HISTORY *of* MEDICAL MIRACLES *and the* LIVES BEHIND THEM

Harry L. Munsinger, J.D., Ph.D.

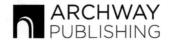

Archway Publishing books may be ordered through booksellers or by contacting:

Archway Publishing
1663 Liberty Drive
Bloomington, IN 47403
www.archwaypublishing.com
844-669-3957

ISBN: 978-1-6657-3139-3 (sc)
ISBN: 978-1-6657-3140-9 (e)

Library of Congress Control Number: 2022918456

Print information available on the last page.

Archway Publishing rev. date: 10/20/2022

Contents

Preface

Ancient Egyptian Medicine

Early Egyptian physicians believed human diseases were caused by angry gods and prescribed magic, mysticism, and rituals to cure illnesses.[1] They thought evil spirits blocked vessels in the body that carry blood, air, semen, mucus, and tears to various organs, causing disease and death. Egyptian physicians used laxatives to unblock the digestive system and prayers to open blood flow to the brain and body. They believed the heart was the center of all life-giving channels, but confused arteries, veins, the intestinal tract, and nerves because Egyptian physicians didn't understand human anatomy. They believed that diseases are caused by angry gods and that incantations, aromas, prayers to statues of the gods, and live animal offerings would cure patients' illnesses. Ancient religious rituals may have actually made some patients feel better due to the placebo effect because believing that prayers to angry gods can cure illness releases natural opioids in the brain that relieve pain.[2] Early Chinese physicians developed a different theory to explain human illness.

Ancient Chinese Medicine

Early Chinese medicine was based on Confucian philosophy and organized the causes of illnesses around polar opposites such as hot-cold, wet-dry, and light-dark, and cycles such as summer, fall, winter, and spring or birth, growth, and death. These primitive Chinese medical theories were based on superstition rather than science and used the complementary concepts of yin and yang to explain sickness and health.[3] Chinese doctors believed vital energy flowed through veins that connect to different organs and that qi, a vital life force, flows through the body and maintains health, but can cause disease if it becomes unbalanced by changes in yin and yang. They treated illness by attempting to restore the balance between internal organs and the external elements of earth, fire, water, wood, and metal by prescribing rituals, dietary changes, exercise, and bathing.

Men and women were treated differently by early Chinese doctors. A sick Chinese male could be examined personally by a doctor, who would touch the patient's skin, palpate his organs, and ask him questions. In contrast, when a Chinese woman fell ill, a doctor had to communicate about her illness through a male family member and use a "doctor's lady" (a female statue) to learn the location of her symptoms. A Chinese doctor was forbidden to touch or observe a naked female patient, so a male family member would point to the location of her pain on a "doctor's lady" and describe her symptoms.[4] Chinese physicians used four procedures to diagnose an illness: looking, listening, smelling, and touching. Centuries passed before physicians began to apply science to the study of sickness and health, but once they did, the practice of medicine began improving and led to more effective treatments for diseases.

The Dawn of Scientific Medicine

The ancient Greek physician Hippocrates, who practiced medicine around 400 BC, believed human illnesses are caused by natural factors and could be cured by surgery or proper medical treatment rather than prayer and magic.[5] His scientific approach to disease was extended by Galen, another Greek physician who lived and worked in the Roman Empire around AD 160.[6] In the sixteenth century, Andres Vesalius began the systematic study of the human anatomy;[7] and a century later, William Harvey demonstrated how blood circulates in the human body.[8] Antonie van Leeuwenhoek created advanced magnifying lenses and founded the field of microbiology because of his curiosity.[9] At the end of the eighteenth century, Edward

Jenner discovered a vaccine for smallpox after he noticed that milkmaids who had contracted cowpox were immune to smallpox.[10] During the nineteenth century, general anesthesia, sterile surgery, the germ theory of disease, and X-rays were developed by William Morton,[11] Joseph Lister,[12] Robert Koch,[13] and Wilhelm Roentgen.[14]

Modern Medicine

The golden age of medicine began in the early twentieth century with the extraction of insulin from animal pancreases by Frederick Banting,[15] the discovery of penicillin by Alexander Fleming,[16] and the modeling of DNA by John Watson and Francis Crick.[17] In the twenty-first century, teams of scientists from around the world mapped the human genome,[18] and Jennifer Doudna found a way to insert new DNA into a human gene, creating a tool able to change human evolution forever.[19]

Assuming the current path of scientific discovery continues, effective treatments for cancer, dementia, and other life-threatening diseases may be found in the near future. However, there is no assurance research will continue to produce advances in the treatment of human disease. Medical miracles happen in unpredictable ways and require advanced preparation, hard work, and scientific insight. Nature is unpredictable, germs mutate in dangerous ways, and they become resistant to antibiotics, so medical researchers must constantly struggle to maintain human health and advance the treatment of disease.

Chapter 1

---- ✦ ----

EARLY GREEK MEDICINE: HIPPOCRATES

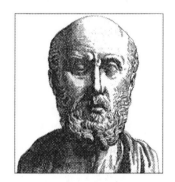

Hippocrates practiced medicine in Greece around 400 BC and was the first physician to show that illnesses are caused by natural factors rather than angry gods. He is called the Father of Medicine, and all modern physicians pledge to follow his ethical example by taking the Hippocratic oath. His most important contributions to medicine were denying that diseases are triggered by evil spirits and proposing that illnesses are caused by natural forces and can be treated by studying symptoms, diagnosing diseases, recording which treatments work for various illnesses, and applying scientific methods to medicine.

Evidence about Greek medicine before Hippocrates comes from ancient writings and fossilized human remains, which show the effects of diseases and treatments administered by early physicians. Prior to Hippocrates, the diagnosis and treatment of diseases were based on religious rituals rather than careful observation and scientific thinking.[20] The number of priest-physicians and surgeons practicing in ancient Greece is difficult to estimate because no accurate historical records are available. Historians have assumed that small Greek towns, which contained fewer than two thousand souls, probably had no physicians available to care for sick and elderly patients because early Greek doctors practiced in large cities such as Athens.[21] A few ancient Greek physicians traveled around the countryside, practicing medicine in villages and small towns, but most preferred to work in cities where they could maintain an office and see patients near their homes rather than having to travel in all kinds of weather over poorly maintained roads to visit their patients in distant areas. Greek physicians practiced medicine and surgery.

Ancient Surgery

Operations were performed by ancient Greek surgeons using instruments made of flint, stone, or shell, making the surgical operations dangerous and painful. Early Greek surgeons amputated damaged or diseased areas of the body by cutting out injured or diseased tissue, sawing off limbs, or drilling into the skull in an effort to cure a sick patient. Ancient Greek surgeons believed illnesses were caused by evil spirits being trapped in the patient's head, so they may have cut a hole in the skull to allow the harmful spirits to escape. Patients who suffered from bleeding and pressure on the brain might have been helped by these dangerous brain operations, but for most patients, they were painful and deadly. We know a few patients survived these primitive brain operations because ancient skulls have been found that show a surgical hole in their skull, which had begun to fill with new bone before the patient died.

Ancient Greek priest-physicians practiced medicine by appealing to their gods for cures and performing religious rituals to cure diseases and stop epidemics. Priests, physicians, midwives, exorcists, bonesetters, and surgeons offered advice and treatments intended to restore a patient's health, but priest-physicians were most popular among the public because appealing to the gods for treatments was less painful than surgery and most of the time just as effective. Priest-physicians often worked in healing temples, which were analogous to modern hospitals, without antiseptic procedures and sterile operating rooms.[22]

Healing Temples

Ancient Greek priest-physicians practiced medicine in healing temples where patients were required to fast before being admitted. Once inside, a patient was told of prior cures to convince him or her that the rituals actually worked. Then the patient was bathed and asked to make an offering to the temple god; if the offering passed muster, the patient was admitted and placed in a bed in a large open room. Hypnotic drugs were administered to produce vivid dreams, which the physician-priest used in planning the treatment for the patient. Some patients actually got better, and the cure was attributed to the gods and the physician's skill. More often, there was no cure, and the patient was blamed for the poor outcome. The priest-physician would accuse the patient of neglecting to do something critical to the cure, absolving himself of responsibility for failure.

While in the temple, patients followed a hygienic routine of eating nourishing food, sleeping, relaxing, bathing, and exercising, which probably helped some recover from their illnesses. Priest-physicians recorded symptoms associated with the illnesses they encountered and studied outcomes so they could predict who would likely recover and who would probably die. But early Greek priest-physicians had little understanding of the diseases they were treating or how to cure them. Amputations were common in the ancient world when a surgeon recognized that an arm, hand, leg, or foot was so seriously damaged or infected it needed to be removed to save the person's life. Surgeons used morphine and alcohol to relieve pain; and they used honey, beer, yeast, oil, dates, figs, onions, garlic, and flaxseeds to fight infections. However, there is little evidence these ancient remedies were effective in avoiding or curing illnesses. Perhaps these ancient patients received some relief from the placebo effect, but early medical practices often did more harm than good.

Early patient care changed for the better when Hippocrates began practicing a primitive form of scientific medicine; he studied diseases systematically, recorded which treatments cured illnesses, and applied systematic procedures to the study of disease.

Hippocrates

What historians know about Hippocrates is derived from writings by him and his followers although some of these manuscripts were written decades after he died. As a result, there are disagreements about his early life because ancient biographers who wrote centuries after Hippocrates's death did not always record accurate information about him. He was most likely born in August 460 BC on the Greek island of Cos, located in the southeastern section of the Aegean Sea near modern Turkey. The most reliable biographical facts about him are contained in two manuscripts believed to have been written by his son Thessalus and Hippocrates himself. Other reliable information about this remarkable ancient physician can be found in the Hippocratic Corpus, a collection of manuscripts stored in the library at Alexandria, which contain notes about his life and medical teachings compiled while he lived and for more than two hundred years after his death.[23]

He is mentioned in Plato's dialogue, *Protagoras*, written about 430 BC. Hippocrates studied medicine with his father, who was a successful Greek physician and left the island of Cos to practice medicine in the larger cities of Greece when he was around thirty. Historians believe he grew up in a family that included his mother, Praxithea; his grandmother, Phainarete; his grandfather, Hippocrates; his father, Heracleides; and his brother, Soranus. Hippocrates was probably disciplined and tutored during childhood by family slaves, who taught him history, diction, and how to tell stories. Records left by early Greek historians suggest young Hippocrates probably played with tops, balls, toy animals, and participated in games such as hide-and-seek, tug-of-war, leapfrog, and blindman's bluff, which were common among Greek children at the time.

Early Education

At around seven years of age, Hippocrates would have been placed under the care of an older slave who walked with him to school in the morning and accompanied him home at night to ensure the boy's safety. Greek primary education lasted nine years; and pupils attended classes in physical education, reading, writing, and spelling. Only Greek boys were sent to school, and they were required to read aloud before the teacher to improve their enunciation and expression.[24] Boys learned to write with a pen and ink on papyrus, an early form of paper developed by Egyptians and imported into Greece. In addition to reading, writing, and physical education, Hippocrates probably studied poetry, music, singing, and how to play a musical instrument such as the flute. Greek education was designed to produce men who could participate in the affairs of the community and provide leadership for the Greek city-states. Teachers were paid by their students and had absolute authority over them. Discipline could include corporal punishment if the offense was serious.

At age sixteen, the sons of wealthy Greek parents entered higher education at a gymnasium school taught by philosophers such as Plato or Aristotle. Hippocrates is believed to have attended a gymnasium on Cos, where he learned to swim, ride, wrestle, and box in addition to mastering languages and philosophy. Greek boys were required to participate in sports to improve and maintain their physical health. Hippocrates probably learned to throw a spear similar to those used in the Greek army because young men were expected to defend their city if it was attacked. Boys typically graduated from a gymnasium school at eighteen and then served two years in the Greek army.[25] Because Hippocrates lived on an island, it's unlikely he served in the Greek army because troops were maintained only by large Greek city-states such as Sparta or Athens. After graduation, wealthy Greek boys would learn a trade or apprentice in a profession such as medicine, law, or the priesthood.

Medical Education

Historians believe Hippocrates studied medicine under the direction of his father, who was a respected physician. Before Hippocrates, Greek medicine was based mainly on superstition rather than science, but he changed medical thinking by arguing that diseases are caused by natural forces and can be cured by surgery or medicines rather than religious rituals. Greek medical students were apprenticed to a practicing physician and attended centers of medical teaching located in healing temples. An important medical temple was located on the island of Cos, and medical students were admitted to these facilities for a fee to study medicine and surgery. There was no standard course of study for a Greek medical student. Instead, they served as assistants to physicians, learning to practice medicine through an apprenticeship.[26]

Medical students accompanied their mentors while they were seeing patients and acquired knowledge in the healing arts and surgery by assisting them as they treated sick individuals. Medical students were required to read medical texts as part of their education. Hippocrates recommended that Greek physicians carefully observe symptoms, systematically collect a medical history, think about the causes of a patient's illness, search for ways to treat diseases, and dutifully record treatments that worked in a notebook. Greek philosophers such as Plato and Empedocles discussed their ideas about nature and science with Hippocrates and other Greek physicians, helping them apply logic and scientific thinking to the study of disease. There was no state supervision of doctors or priests in ancient Greece, so patients were free to choose the type of care they preferred. Greek patients often selected religious cures rather than scientific treatments because they were cheaper and less painful than surgery.

Ancient Greek treatments for broken bones and joint dislocations were similar to modern medical practices, but Greek physicians lacked accurate knowledge of anatomy and the structure and function of internal organs, so complex surgery was only recommended as a last resort when other treatments had failed and the patient was near death. Anatomical knowledge increased after Aristotle started dissecting animals, but remained primitive until the sixteenth century when Vesalius began dissecting human cadavers and producing detailed anatomical drawings of the human body.[27] Hippocrates pioneered the scientific study of medicine and surgery, and that's the reason he's called the "Father of Medicine." He traveled to Greek islands in the Aegean Sea, Greek cities on the mainland, and to Egypt and Libya during his long life to learn how other physicians practiced medicine. During his travels, Hippocrates studied the methods and practices of the foreign doctors he encountered, trying to learn new and effective treatments for various diseases. He recommended that physicians treat the whole person rather than focus on a disease in isolation and prescribed rest, a balanced diet, bathing, and exercise for the treatment of many diseases. These simple restorative treatments sometimes worked because of the body's natural healing abilities. Students flocked to Hippocrates to learn better medical practices than were available elsewhere.

Medical Students

Hippocrates believed anyone who wanted to be a physician must love the profession, acquire the necessary training, and be disciplined enough to practice under difficult conditions. Physicians and surgeons were respected in ancient Greece because people hoped they could keep them healthy. Greek city-states hired physicians to treat soldiers, and a few Greek governments offered free medical services to the poor. However, most ancient Greek physicians worked in private practices treating patients for a fee, so wealthy individuals enjoyed better medical care than their poor peers. Ancient Greek physicians usually saw patients at the office, but would make home visits to important individuals or patients too ill to get out of bed. Busy doctors employed medical students as assistants to help them treat patients and make diagnoses, perform surgeries, and prescribe herbal medicines to treat illnesses. Ancient Greek physicians specialized in different branches of medicine, including surgery, vision, diseases of women, and podiatry.

Scientific Medicine

Hippocrates was the first physician to develop a systematic approach to medicine, and for centuries after his death, his writings formed the foundation of medical practice. Hippocrates wrote, "All [diseases] are alike divine, for each has its own nature, and each disease has a natural cause—and without a natural cause none arise."[28] His insistence that all diseases were caused by natural forces gradually shifted European medical practice from superstition and ignorance toward the scientific study of diseases. Physicians in other cultures continued to rely on magical incantations and mystical procedures to cure diseases they attributed to evil spirits, vengeful ancestors, or angry gods long after the Greeks and Romans began practicing scientific medicine.

Hippocrates taught medical students to record the symptoms of diseases, study their natural course, and search for medicines or surgical procedures to alleviate suffering and help patients recover their health. He recommended studying the outcomes of illness to better understand the disease and treat patients effectively. Hippocrates taught medical students how to collect a comprehensive medical history, including asking the patient about sleep habits, employment, exposure to others who were ill, and prior personal illnesses. He recommended that physicians look carefully at a patient's eyes, skin, ears, and forehead; listen to their chest, heart, and lungs for signs of disease; and then diagnose a patient's illness and prescribe the proper treatment to cure the sickness.[29] Hippocrates not only studied and taught, but he also practiced medicine every day by seeing sick patients.

Hippocrates's Medical Practice

A typical day for Hippocrates started with visits to patients who were too sick to get out of bed. He treated them in their homes or at a healing temple, which was analogous to a modern hospital, except the facilities were primitive. Hippocrates often observed that patients developed a fever for several days, but when the fever went away, the patient recovered. He didn't understand why this happened but concluded that when a fever disappeared, that was a positive sign and the patient was likely to recover and live. Hippocrates knew that patients who experience recurring fevers rarely recovered, but sometimes they could live with the chronic condition for years. Modern physicians believe these patients likely contracted some form of malaria, which was common in Greece at the time. Hippocrates separated diseases into two classes, which he called external and internal.

Illnesses of the skin or eyes, which could be seen with the eyes or felt with the hands, he called external diseases while internal diseases could only be inferred by observing their symptoms. Hippocrates asked patients suffering from internal diseases to describe the pain and other symptoms they experienced so he could diagnose the problem and prescribe a treatment. He believed sick patients should not get out of bed except to visit the toilet and they should be kept warm and comfortable. In contrast, modern physicians encourage their surgery patients to get out of bed and move around as soon as possible after their operation to regain strength and mobility. Hippocrates recommended that patients drink adequate water, live in a house with good ventilation, eat healthy food, and take mild enemas to ensure they had regular bowel movements. He believed telling a patient the likely course of the illness was important to gain their trust and raise the patient's spirits so they would more likely survive the disease.

Rules of Health and Disease

During his life, Hippocrates compiled basic rules concerning illness:

1. People who are overweight are likely to die sooner than thin people.
2. Among old people, it is normal to see coughs, joint pains, poor eyesight, dullness of hearing, and cataracts.
3. Slight sweating during a fever is a bad sign.
4. Sensitivity to touch is a bad sign when a patient is ill.
5. In an acute disease, it is difficult to predict death or recovery.
6. During a fever, it is bad for the patient to feel chilled externally, burn inside, and be thirsty.

7. Most fevers last about fourteen days, and the patient then recovers or dies.
8. Deep sleep signals the end of a crisis while disturbed sleep with pain is an indication that the patient is not improving.
9. Drowsiness in a patient is usually a bad sign.
10. Frequent pain in the heart of an older person often signals death.
11. Constant noise in the ears is a sign of an acute disease.

Guide to Health

Among his many manuscripts, Hippocrates wrote *A Regimen for Health*, which was an everyday guide to healthy living. He advised patients to exercise, eat a well-balanced diet, care for their teeth, and maintain good habits. Hippocrates recommended running or wrestling to maintain fitness and suggested that moderate exercise interspersed with rest was best for older persons. He advised against exercising immediately after eating, suggesting it would interfere with digestion. These recommendations are similar to modern doctors' suggestions for health—exercise moderately to avoid becoming weak and flabby and eat a healthy diet, but don't overdo it. Hippocrates knew a balanced diet is essential for health and believed an appropriate diet depends on the individual's age, habits, job, and season of the year.

He recommended moist foods for young infants and sick adults because they are easy to digest and suggested people eat less in the summer and more in the winter. He also gave advice about weight loss, recommending that eating boiled and baked foods was better than consuming foods fried in fats when trying to lose weight. Hippocrates suggested children eat fruits, vegetables, and meats from animals fed milk, grass, and grain. He recommended that adults drink wine to maintain good health, and many modern adults heartily agree. Modern dieticians recommend individuals eat a diet containing green and yellow vegetables, fruits, potatoes, milk, cheese, meat, bread, cereals, and butter. Hippocrates didn't know vitamins are important for good health, but he was wise enough to recognize that a variety of foods helped people stay healthy. He wrote that skin, hair, and nails are important because they protect the body from injury and infection, regulate temperature, and eliminate waste. Hippocrates prescribed daily bathing in warm water for his patients and suggested using a sponge to clean the skin because he believed warm baths soothe a patient, wash away waste, relieve fatigue, and encourage healing of the skin. Hippocrates's theory of health assumed that human diseases were caused by imbalances in body fluids, which he called humors.

The Four Humors

Early Greek philosophers and physicians were interested in the origins of all things and developed theories about how everything worked, including how the body functioned. Hippocrates proposed that imbalances among four body fluids cause most human diseases.[30] His text, *On the Nature of Man*, listed these fluids as yellow bile, black bile, blood, and phlegm (known to later physicians as the four humors). Hippocrates believed a person would enjoy good health when these humors were balanced and would fall ill when one humor dominated the others. He believed the four humors could become unbalanced through prolonged exposure to excessively hot, cold, wet, or dry conditions. Hippocrates recommended that medical treatments focus on a patient's mind and body and that physicians pay attention to objective symptoms as well as how the patient feels and what he or she says when diagnosing a disease. He focused on treating acute illnesses and didn't worry much about the chronic conditions of aging, believing they were a natural part of life. Hippocrates was a gifted physician and teacher who attracted students from all over the ancient world; he taught them how to observe and record symptoms to diagnose and treat illnesses.

He taught his students to search for and record surgical procedures and herbal medicines that helped a patient recover and admonished doctors to "do no harm." Hippocrates recommended that physicians record what parts of the body were affected by different diseases, study the course of swelling, note instances of vomiting, evacuations of the bowels, coughing, thirst, hunger, dreams, pains, and the patient's ability to understand simple concepts. He emphasized the diagnosis of disease by observing specific bodily conditions. Even today, physicians collect a patient's medical history to diagnose illnesses, understand a patient's problem, and prescribe a cure.

Hippocrates studied fevers in detail to understand their causes and cures because they were frequent in early Greece. Many of the cases described by Hippocrates involved fevers, which modern physicians believe were caused by parasites, bacteria, or viruses. However, ancient Greek physicians could only describe, categorize, and speculate about the causes and cures of the fevers they observed because they had no microscopes or other advanced instruments available to study germs.

Fever

Hippocrates believed body temperature was an important symptom of many diseases, and he paid special attention to the pattern of fever and whether it was acute, recurring, or chronic. Since he had no measuring instrument to record a patient's temperature accurately, Hippocrates studied external signs of fevers such as skin color, body heat, urine color, reported pain, and the patient's mood. Based on his study of malarial fevers, Hippocrates discovered there were critical periods in illnesses, and these periods could be survived if proper precautions were taken and effective treatments prescribed.[31] He recognized that fever was a reliable symptom of many diseases and knew fevers often appeared among a significant part of the population during epidemics when many people fell ill at the same time. Hippocrates speculated that something was spreading the disease from one person to another, causing fever and death, but he had no understanding of germs or exactly what was causing an epidemic. He was curious about everything and tried to develop theories about what was happening to patients with different symptoms.

Hippocrates sometimes found that a fever would develop in one patient and not spread to others; but more often, he observed that when one person became sick and developed a fever, the illness and fever spread to others who had been in contact with the sick patient. He encouraged his medical students to follow the course of a fever, record its pattern, and observe breathing and perspiration to diagnose the underlying disease. Hippocrates concluded that a fever that progressed rapidly was most dangerous to the life of a patient. He also knew that some fevers disappear on their own, so he tried to diagnose illnesses and record their outcomes in order to understand the course of a disease and predict how likely the patient was to survive. Hippocrates knew nothing about parasites, bacteria, or viruses, but he did advise physicians that the characteristics of a fever offered objective evidence of specific illnesses and that the course of fever could often predict the outcome of different diseases. He studied a plague that killed thousands in ancient Athens and attempted to stop it by burning fires in the city to purify the air. The people of Athens believed he had saved them, but modern physicians are not certain what stopped the plague.

The Plague of Athens

Sanitation in Greek cities was terrible. There were no sewers or regular supplies of potable water, and the streets were piled high with garbage. Epidemics were rampant, and childhood mortality high among the ancient Greeks. Between 430 and 426 BC, Athens suffered two serious outbreaks of a mysterious disease that killed a high percentage of those who contracted the illness.[32] Based on recorded symptoms of the disease, modern physicians don't believe it was a bubonic plague. Instead, they have speculated that the epidemic was caused by measles, smallpox, typhus, or influenza. Since he knew nothing of germs, Hippocrates proposed that epidemics were the result of imbalances among four humors caused by a mismatch between the individual and his or her environment. He believed patients needed to eat a healthy diet, exercise, and get adequate sleep to prevent illness and prescribed purges, fasting, and emetics to balance the four humors once a person became sick. Hippocrates didn't understand that diseases could be transmitted from one person to another by breathing, touching, or drinking contaminated water, and had little knowledge of public sanitation. Moreover, his theory of humors didn't help much in understanding how to treat diseases or stop plagues.

The problem with Hippocrates's theory was that if a person's health depended on individual behaviors and imbalances of humors, how could he explain why people who were behaving in different ways became ill with similar symptoms at the same time during an epidemic? Before Hippocrates, the answer would have been that the deaths were caused by an angry god, as suggested by Homer in the *Odyssey*. Hippocrates rejected the idea that angry gods cause disease and speculated instead that epidemics were caused by bad air because this was the only factor common to children, adults, and the aged. He was on the right track but didn't have the tools necessary to see the germs causing different diseases. According to legend, Hippocrates stopped the plague of Athens by burning large bonfires in the city to purify the air, believing whatever was causing the plague was in the air and fire would drive it away. The bonfires probably had little effect on the plague, but it did disappear, as epidemics often do after a majority of the population contracts the illness and dies or develops immunity. Hippocrates also recommended that medical students study anatomy as part of their medical education, especially if they intended to be surgeons.

Anatomy and Surgery

Hippocrates wrote that pathology is the study of changes in the body caused by disease and advised physicians to learn the anatomical structure of a human body so they could differentiate normal from abnormal organs. Modern doctors look at samples of a patient's blood and tissue and analyze them chemically to diagnose many diseases in more sophisticated ways than were available to Hippocrates, who worked with primitive information about the composition of blood and other body fluids. However, even with his limited knowledge of how the human body functions, Hippocrates developed some remarkable medical ideas. He studied the effect of climate on eating, drinking, and digestion. Galen also understood that fluids in the stomach are essential to digestion although he didn't know that the fluids are enzymes that facilitate chemical reactions in the stomach, which produce the energy needed for an organism to live and move. Hippocrates was also a skilled surgeon and taught his students how to perform complex operations.

He performed surgical operations involving cutting, scraping, and sawing to remove diseased tissue or amputate a limb to save a life.[33] Hippocrates taught medical students the various surgical techniques available at the time and recommended they use an assistant to help during an operation and employ good surgical instruments to improve the outcome. However, he had no understanding of germs and the necessity of sterilizing his instruments and hands prior to operating. Hippocrates did recognize that good lighting was important during surgery. He described how to place a silk sheet between a light source, such as the sun, and the site of the operation to eliminate shadows and give the surgeon a better view of the patient's organs during an operation. He taught students how to bandage a wound after surgery to keep it clean, stop bleeding, and aid healing. Hippocrates defined psychiatry and neurology as the study of mood and nervous system disorders.

Psychiatry and Neurology

He wrote that psychiatry and neurology are concerned with a patient's emotional and cognitive problems; believed that pleasure, joy, laughter, sorrow, pain, and grief arise in the brain; and that the normal functioning brain enables seeing, hearing, thinking, and distinguishing good, bad, beauty, and ugliness. Hippocrates wrote that the brain directs other organs of the body by interpreting events in the world and stimulating the body to action. He believed intellect occurred in the brain and that too much heat or humidity caused most abnormal behaviors. Hippocrates proposed that anxiety, depression, and delirium were caused by physical damage to the brain or imbalances among the four humors.

Hippocrates treated persons with mental illnesses in his practice and described one case of a woman who was in despair from losing her husband. She was depressed, refused to eat, and was near death. Hippocrates asked the woman to tell him about her loss and sadness and listened sympathetically. He then counseled her by pointing out that her refusal to eat was affecting the entire family and causing them severe pain. Hippocrates shifted the woman's focus from her own loss to the needs of her children and helped her recover from severe depression and resume a normal life. He emphasized the importance of proper nursing during the recovery of patients and recommended that hospital rooms should be shaded, cool, comfortable, away from the wind, on the ground floor, dark, and visitors should be discouraged. He also studied epileptic seizures systematically rather than ascribing them to angry gods.[34]

For centuries, epileptic seizures were called the "sacred disease" because priest-physicians believed they were caused by angry gods. Hippocrates rejected this explanation and wrote that epileptic seizures were caused by damage to the brain although he didn't know the exact reason they happened. He said that priest-physicians who called epilepsy "sacred" were no more than witch doctors who hid their ignorance behind magic and purification rites that did no good. Hippocrates also collected and studied plants to determine which could be used to treat human diseases.

Early Greek physicians borrowed herbal treatments from Egyptian medicine prior to Hippocrates, but he formulated more effective plant-based remedies through systematic study rather than magical thinking and developed effective cures for a few diseases. He suggested that sick or elderly patients should move to a milder climate to regain their health if they were sensitive to cold. One of his favorite medicines was honey boiled in water because Hippocrates believed it would soften the lungs, alleviate coughing, and act as a mild diuretic. Hippocrates operated a busy and varied medical practice and attracted many students because of his success in treating patients. He treated diseases of the eye and teeth.

Eye Care

Hippocrates believed vision is the most important sense because it produces critical information for brain development and function. He also wrote that careful observation of the eye will reveal a patient's general health. Hippocrates taught his medical students to pay close attention to swelling of the eye, light sensitivity, inflammation, tearing, rapid blinking, and headaches as signs of eye disease. He believed that pain in the eye is often a sign of serious illness and must be taken seriously. Hippocrates said that because the eyes are used daily, they need special care and frequent rest. He recommended that when an individual is doing detailed work, he or she should rest the eyes frequently and suggested that when an individual is ill, the eyes should be used sparingly and the patient should stay in a darkened room. In addition to treating eyes, Hippocrates also fixed teeth.

Dentistry

The skulls of ancient Greeks show their teeth were generally well preserved because their diet contained fruits, vegetables, and meats and they ate few sweets; many died young.[35] Hippocrates had a rudimentary understanding of dentistry and recommended that diseased teeth be extracted to keep a patient from becoming ill and dying. He recognized that young children suffer mild pain and fever when growing new teeth, but believed the process was natural and told parents their children would be fine and not to worry about it. He understood that tooth decay was related to diet and suggested people clean their teeth daily and avoid sweet foods because they contributed to tooth decay. He didn't understand that the combination of bacteria in the mouth and carbohydrates causes tooth decay, but he knew that proper diet and cleaning help maintain healthy teeth.[36] Hippocrates knew nothing about adding fluoride to drinking water to strengthen teeth because its benefit was not discovered until the twentieth century. He developed a code of ethics for physicians that evolved into the modern Hippocratic Oath.

The Hippocratic Oath

It's unlikely Hippocrates actually wrote the oath that bears his name. It was probably drafted by later physicians who were inspired by his ethical treatment of patients. Hippocrates emphasized patient privacy, caring for life, and doing no harm. He stated that a doctor should not divulge information learned during treatment because that could damage doctor-patient trust, and he refused to prescribe poison for terminally ill patients, saying the task of the physician was to save lives, not end them. Hippocrates recommended physicians seek advice from colleagues and avoid trying to enhance their reputation by making false claims. He admitted he didn't know how to cure many diseases and strived to be honest in his dealings with patients and other physicians. His oath sets out the ideals of modern medical practice.[37]

The Modern Hippocratic Oath

I swear to fulfill this covenant:
I will respect science.
I apply all required measures.
Medicine is art and science.
I respect privacy.
I treat a human being.
I prevent disease.
I preserve traditions.

According to fragmentary historical records, Hippocrates probably died in 361 BC at the age of ninety. Following his death, Greek medicine stagnated, and almost four hundred years passed before another Greek physician comparable to Hippocrates appeared. His name was Claudius Galenus and was known as "Galen."

Chapter 2

---- ✦ ----

EARLY ROMAN MEDICINE: GALEN

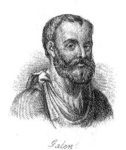

Galen

Galen believed experience is the source of all knowledge and paid special attention to medical treatments that worked. He studied anatomy by performing public dissections of living animals and demonstrated brain functions by pressing on different areas of exposed animal brains, causing temporary blindness or paralysis. Galen was a physician to a school of gladiators; treated their wounds with oil, herbs, and wine to prevent infections; and used the content of dreams to diagnose illnesses. Later, he became a court physician to Emperor Marcus Aurelius and treated his family. For centuries, Galen's writings were considered the Holy Bible of medicine and could not be contradicted. However, Galen made mistakes about human anatomy because he based his writings on animal dissections.

Galen was born in Pergamum, a Greek city on the Adriatic coast near present-day Turkey in September AD 129. His father was a wealthy architect who hired philosophers to teach Galen geometry, mathematics, grammar, logic, and Greek.[38] Galen received an excellent education before he was apprenticed to a physician to study medicine. He read widely in medical texts and studied the structure of muscles, bones, veins, and arteries by dissecting living animals. In the middle of his medical education, Galen self-diagnosed a serious illness in himself, which happens often among young medical students.

Medical Student's Syndrome

Along with many other students over the centuries, Galen fell victim to "medical student's syndrome."[39] He developed intestinal pain while studying diseases of the digestive tract and self-diagnosed an abscess in his gut, which he believed might be fatal although it was probably an upset stomach. Even today, self-diagnosis of a serious illness is common among young medical students after they learn the symptoms of a new disease. After his self-diagnosis, Galen had a dream telling him to cut an artery between his right index and middle fingers to cure his stomach abscess. He immediately cut the artery he had dreamed about, gave up eating fresh fruit, began exercising, and his stomach pain disappeared. Modern physicians are not certain what cured Galen's stomach pain, but giving up fresh fruit and exercising were more likely cures than bloodletting. Galen learned to mix herbal medicines to treat different illnesses and acquired medical knowledge from many physicians. He never adhered to any medical philosophy, preferring to borrow from any theory that seemed to work. The three competing medical philosophies at that time were called empiricists, rationalists, and methodists.

Empiricists

Empirical physicians believed that experience was the source of all knowledge, paid attention to medical treatments that worked, and recorded them in manuscripts so future physicians would know how to cure the disease when it occurred in another patient. Effective treatment might be the result of a happy accident, a lucky guess, or based on a dream; but for the treatment to be valid, empiricists believed it needed to work most of the time. A few recoveries were not adequate evidence that a treatment worked because ancient physicians knew patients sometimes recovered on their own without treatment. Galen accepted the empiricist assertion that all knowledge comes from experience and believed that physicians should observe and record patients' symptoms, make a diagnosis based on symptoms, and select the best treatment for the disease.[40] He was an empiricist but also paid some attention to the rationalist theory of medicine because logic and deduction appealed to him philosophically.

Rationalists

Rational physicians based their medical practices on theories about the causes of disease and deductions from these theories. Galen used deductive reasoning in his medical practice and studied rationalist theories about the human body and the causes and courses of disease, but was not a strict adherent to the idea that a physician could diagnose illnesses deductively and select the proper treatment based on theory alone. He preferred to rely primarily on personal experience and observation of a patient to diagnose diseases and develop therapies that worked rather than relying on theory and deduction. Galen rejected the methodist philosophy of medicine out of hand because he concluded it was absurd.

Methodists

The methodist school of medicine believed diseases are caused by atoms being too tightly compressed or dispersed within the human body, rejected the study of anatomy, and claimed a physician could be trained in less than six months using their method. Galen called methodist physicians "quacks" and would have nothing to do with them. Before Galen, many Roman physicians believed diseases were caused by angry gods, and the best treatment was for a patient to make an offering to the Roman gods of medicine and health. Galen rejected this view of medicine although it was popular throughout the Roman Empire. Aesculapius, the Roman god of medicine, and Hygeia, the Roman goddess of health, were believed to have the power to cure diseases; and many temples were erected so patients could pray for the recovery of their health.[41]

Galen rejected the idea that illnesses are caused by angry gods and that magical rituals could cure diseases. He believed illnesses can be cured by applying physical treatments, herbal medicines, and surgical procedures. Galen did acknowledge that magical potions or religious rituals occasionally made patients feel better, but he didn't know why. Today, physicians believe patients sometimes feel better because of the placebo effect, which happens when a person believes a treatment will work and their faith releases opioid-like substances in their brain, which reduce pain. Galen also accepted Hippocrates's theory of humors, associating them with phlegmatic, sanguine, choleric, and melancholic temperaments. He refused to follow the teachings of any one school of medicine, borrowed from many and accepted any treatment that worked.

In AD 157, Galen returned to Pergamum after traveling through parts of the Roman Empire studying different medical techniques. He was offered an opportunity to treat serious wounds when he became a physician to a band of gladiators.

Physician to Gladiators

Gladiatorial games were funded by wealthy citizens for public entertainment, and Greek cities had a long tradition of employing skilled physicians to treat them. Being hired by the city of Pergamum to treat gladiators was an honor for the young physician.[42] Gladiator games began as entertainment at the funerals of Roman aristocrats, but gradually, the games became more spectacular and were staged for general public entertainment. In Rome, gladiatorial games were sponsored by the emperor and staged near the end of each year. Greek and Roman cities also sponsored boxing and wrestling matches in which fingers were broken, limbs dislocated, and eyes bloodied or gouged. Roman citizens liked blood sports, and fights to the death were common.

Gladiators were generally managed by a high priest who bought and trained them. Pairs of gladiators from the same group fought each other, and the Roman crowd decided whether the loser survived or died. Disobedient slaves and criminals were often sold as gladiators for punishment. Gladiatorial contests could be fought to the death although the priest who owned them preferred to spare his men because they were expensive to purchase, train, and maintain. The crowd's decision was seldom ignored, however. Gladiators who fought bravely were generally spared to fight another day, and most gladiators fought several battles before being killed in the arena or dying from a serious infection days after they were wounded. A few lucky gladiators lived to retire, but most died young. They fought according to rules of engagement enforced by a referee. Gladiators were expected to fight bravely and hope for victory but were not supposed to wound or kill an opponent unnecessarily. A contest usually lasted about fifteen minutes before one of the gladiators won.[43] Roman gladiators were fed fava beans and boiled barley to help them accumulate fat, which was believed to prevent infections if they were wounded.

Galen treated gladiatorial wounds with surgery and a mixture of oil, herbs, and wine, which he believed facilitated healing and curbed infection. He cleaned and sutured transverse thigh and arm wounds to reconnect the severed muscle and skin, but if the wound was vertical, Galen believed it was sufficient to bind the injury and allow the muscle and skin to heal on their own. Galen criticized physicians who only stitched the skin over transverse muscle wounds, saying that transverse muscle cuts must be sewn together so they will heal properly and function. Once the wound was stitched, he soaked linen in wine, olive oil, and herbs before applying the cloth directly to the gladiator's injury and continued adding wine to the linen to keep it moist. The alcohol and acidity in wine may have inhibited infections when applied for extended intervals. Galen knew nothing of germs but believed keeping a wound moist with wine encouraged healing and discouraged infection.

He believed that thread made in Gaul was best for suturing wounds but used silk if thread from Gaul was not available. He also recommended using strips of animal gut for sutures. Galen noted that when a gladiator was wounded in the heart, he invariably died though it might take days. Two gladiators died during Galen's first year as their physician, but his predecessor had lost sixteen gladiators during a similar interval. His tenure treating gladiators ended in AD 161 when Galen left for Rome. He studied different diets as he traveled through the Roman Empire, hoping to discover correlations between human health and eating habits. He noticed that Egyptians ate large quantities of pistachios but could discover no beneficial effect of the diet on their health. Galen attributed the development of elephantiasis to eating donkey meat (modern physicians know that the hardening of skin and swelling of the arms, legs, hands, and feet are caused by parasitic larvae passed to humans by mosquitoes). He believed the disease could be cured by bleeding and ingesting snake venom. Galen walked to Rome when he was thirty-two, making the journey with a group of travelers to avoid attacks by bandits.

Rome

During his travels to Rome, Galen collected ingredients for herbal medicines, bought plants from an Indian camel caravan, and purchased copper and silver from mine managers. He sailed to the islands of Cyprus and Lemnos to collect samples of earth from those places because ancient physicians believed the dirt could cure snakebite. When Galen arrived in Rome, he found that the city was overcrowded, unsanitary, and plagued by epidemics. Rome had two advantages over most European cities: abundant freshwater and grain from Egypt that kept Roman citizens clean, hydrated, and nourished so they could ward off some diseases naturally. Only common Roman citizens were eligible to receive free allotments of Egyptian grain while patricians were generally wealthy enough to afford a nourishing diet for themselves. When the Tiber River flooded every few years, it usually contaminated the water supply and caused an epidemic that killed thousands of Romans. Citizens also caught infections in public baths.

Wealthy Romans bathed once a day in public baths or at home.[44]

Bathing was considered a civilized luxury in Rome, but the baths spread disease because Roman authorities didn't know they should disinfect the warm bathwater with chlorine to kill infectious germs. Sick patients were typically bathed around 3:00 p.m. daily in the public baths, and the heated water was an ideal medium for microbes to grow and infect others. Galen warned his patients not to expose open wounds to public bathwater because that could cause infections. Diseases were also spread by flies, mosquitoes, contaminated water, or airborne particles throughout Rome. Malaria was endemic in the city and reached a peak every year during the late summer months when mosquitos were everywhere. Conditions for producing mosquitoes were nearly ideal in Rome because there was abundant stagnant water in lakes and ponds near the Tiber River and the climate was mild. Romans believed the higher ground was healthier than lower areas near the river, probably reflecting the higher incidence of malarial mosquitoes in low wet areas near the Tiber River. Galen paid special attention to "fevers," which he believed could give reliable clues for diagnosing different diseases.[45]

Fever

Galen's description of "fever" is similar to the symptoms of malaria, which includes recurring bouts of temperature, sweating, digestive problems, muscle tension, dizziness, headache, chills, and vomiting. In addition to malaria, Roman citizens suffered epidemics of smallpox, which was fatal in about 30 percent of cases, and tuberculosis, a wasting disease characterized by coughing and usually death years later. Death from tuberculosis was most prevalent among younger Roman adults, perhaps because older citizens had already contracted the disease, survived, and were immune. The average life expectancy of a Roman citizen was around twenty-five years due to high infant mortality and recurring epidemics caused by poor sanitation and infectious diseases. The contrast between Rome and Pergamum must have been stark for Galen. Pergamum had a total population of around one hundred twenty thousand while Rome's population was estimated to have been over one million during Galen's lifetime, and the city teemed with diseases.[46]

Roman Medicine

Medical specialization was common in Rome, with many physicians limiting their practice to eyes, ears, gynecology, or surgery. Galen practiced general medicine and surgery in Rome. His first important patient was Eudemus, a sixty-three-year-old friend who fell ill soon after Galen arrived in Rome. He asked Galen what he should do after he suffered chills for three days and continued to feel ill. Galen diagnosed quartan fever based on the recurring temperature he experienced every three days. Modern physicians believe the fever was probably caused by a strain of malaria common in Rome at the time. Galen believed fever was a dangerous symptom and could be fatal, so he took his friend's illness seriously. While taking a medical history, Galen learned that Eudemus had been prescribed theriac by another physician and the fevers had appeared shortly after the initial dose of that remedy. Galen recommended that his friend stop taking theriac and see if he felt better.

Other physicians who examined Eudemus decided his condition was hopeless and abandoned him, but Galen continued to treat Eudemus, predicting that if he stopped taking theriac he would be cured after three more fevers. Galen's prognosis proved correct: Eudemus began to feel better after stopping theriac and recovered in a few weeks. It's not certain what actually cured Eudemus. Possibly the prescribed theriac was sickening him because it contained snake venom and was ingested as an antidote by important people who believed they might be poisoned. Another possibility is that Eudemus recovered because his immune system suppressed his illness and Galen was lucky enough to be his physician at the time.

The study of medicine was popular among wealthy Roman citizens because they wanted to improve their own health and often didn't trust local physicians. Galen was frequently asked to write educational manuscripts for his wealthy Roman patients because they trusted his judgment. He taught them how to dissect animals and took them along when he treated patients. Galen saw himself as a philosopher and didn't accept money for teaching or treating patients because he was independently wealthy due to an inheritance from his father. One of Galen's most important patients was a Roman senator named Flavius Boethus, who considered himself Greek although he was born a Roman citizen.[47] Eudemus praised Galen to Boethus, and the senator said he wanted to meet this skilled physician. Boethus observed many of Galen's dissections, which he performed in the public square before a crowd of interested onlookers.

Animal Dissections

Dissections of live animals appealed to Roman followers of Aristotle, who pioneered the study of anatomy. Aristotle attributed the order and complexity he found in animals to an intelligent creator and believed physicians and philosophers should pay careful attention to evidence and logic when trying to understand nature and the human body. In his own dissections of animals, Galen discovered that Aristotle had made mistakes about anatomy, such as believing intelligence resided in the heart rather than the brain and that the heart had three chambers rather than four, so he became skeptical of what Aristotle had written about anatomy. Galen did follow Aristotle's advice about dissecting animals to learn anatomy because it was illegal to dissect human cadavers.

After 150 BC, Roman law prohibited the dissection of human cadavers, so Galen was forced to dissect animals to learn anatomy.[48] He practiced animal dissections privately before putting on public demonstrations so he could perform the dissections perfectly, generally using live goats, pigs, and monkeys as subjects. Galen considered monkeys to be similar to humans and most helpful for learning about human anatomy. He had macaques and baboons imported from Egypt and West Africa, but preferred macaques for dissection because they had an upright posture, round faces, opposed thumbs, lacked large canine teeth, and were not aggressive. Galen disliked dissecting baboons, which he considered aggressive and dangerous. He also dissected dogs, mice, snakes, cranes, and fish to study comparative anatomy. He didn't dissect insects because they were too small, but he did dissect an elephant. Galen paid particular attention to the structure and function of animal brains in his studies.

Brain Surgery

Galen performed dissections on living animal brains to demonstrate neural functions, describing the procedure as follows: slice through the skin in a single stroke to expose the skull, cut away the top of the skull without damaging the meninx (a membrane surrounding the brain and spinal cord), and cut away the meninx by pulling it off the brain with hooks. He performed these operations in the summer or in a warm room because cold killed the animal while he operated on its brain. After Galen had exposed the living brain, he pressed on various areas and released them to show how he could disable and revive various sensory and perceptual abilities. For example, if he pressed on the anterior ventricle of the brain near the optic nerve, the pressure caused blindness in the animal. Since Galen couldn't dissect humans, he made several anatomical mistakes, such as believing there are two chambers in the human uterus because there are two in some animals. Neither Galen nor any other ancient anatomist understood that blood circulates to the lungs and the body from the heart through arteries and back to the heart through veins. It took until the seventeenth century for William Harvey to discover that the human pulse and blood circulation are caused by contractions of the heart and to understand how blood circulates to the lungs and throughout the body. Harvey found that Galen had made many anatomical mistakes because he studied animals rather than human bodies.

Galen described what he was doing and observing while he dissected animals and had his comments transcribed and published to teach others how to do dissection. Senator Boethus was a generous supporter of Galen's public dissections and invited important friends, including the emperor to view Galen at work. Galen wrote several anatomical manuscripts for Boethus, including *On the Anatomy of Living Animals* and *On the Anatomy of Dead Animals*. In his manuscript *On the Usefulness of Parts*, Galen said all living beings were constructed by a creator who was either an engineer or an artist. He believed there was intelligence behind creation, but not the omnipotent God of the Christians who could bring creatures into existence by fiat. Galen rejected the idea that knowledge could be acquired by faith; he believed logic and evidence would produce a more accurate picture of nature and man than revelation. In a manuscript *On the Doctrines of Hippocrates and Plato*, Galen said they were generally correct. He dedicated several of his texts to Boethus and sent copies of manuscripts with the senator when he left to govern a distant Roman province. Boethus developed such trust in Galen that he asked him to treat his family when they fell ill.[49]

Boethus's Family

Galen cured Boethus's son after the senator asked him to treat the child because he had a rapid pulse. Galen observed the boy's pulse and realized he was not in serious danger but was more likely anxious. He guessed the boy was hiding something in his room, probably food which he was eating when his mother went to the bath. Galen searched the room and discovered food wrapped in a woman's headscarf. He also treated Boethus's wife, who was suffering from an undiagnosed female disease. The woman was being treated by midwives, but Boethus called Galen because she was not improving. Boethus's wife was being treated by removing excess fluids from her body to balance her four humors. The midwife had her lie down in warm sand and smeared her skin with pitch and resin to extract excess fluid from her body, but the treatment was not helping. One day while she was in her bath, Boethus's wife suffered pains similar to childbirth, expelled a large quantity of fluid from her uterus, and fainted. Galen revived her with smelling salts and massaged her hands and feet until she felt better. He told the midwife to stop the drying treatments and gave her boiled honey, diuretic drugs, and laxatives. Galen asked Boethus to entrust his wife's care to him alone and he agreed. The wife gradually improved after expelling the liquid from her uterus. Boethus was impressed with Galen's diagnostic skills and medical abilities after these two successful outcomes.[50] Modern physicians are not certain what illness the senator's wife suffered, but it may have been a pelvic abscess that resolved spontaneously while she was taking a bath. Boethus gave Galen four hundred gold coins as a token of his gratitude and decided to learn medicine from him. Galen left Rome suddenly in AD 166, and at the time, it was assumed he departed because he might be ordered to accompany the emperor on his campaign in the German province. Years later, Galen said he left Rome because a plague was approaching the city and he wanted to avoid it.

Greek physicians believed effective treatments for disease were often revealed in dreams induced by hypnotic drugs given to patients. Galen took dreams seriously, believing they contained messages from a divine spark within every human being.[51] He thought many of his best medical ideas came from dreams, that dreams reflect conditions within the body and could be used to diagnose illnesses. Galen wrote that if a patient dreamed of standing in a pool of blood, that meant he or she suffered from an excess of blood. Dreaming of ice or snow represented an excess of the cold humor phlegm, and if a patient dreamed that his leg had turned to wood, the person was about to become paralyzed. Galen believed in the existence of gods, arguing they must be real because who else could have created such wondrous creatures as humans and given them omens in the form of dreams? He exercised regularly under the direction of a trainer and one day suffered a serious orthopedic injury.

Collarbone Dislocation

Galen went to the gymnasium every day and was in excellent physical condition all his life. During one strenuous exercise session, he dislocated his collarbone. A modern physician would most likely have diagnosed a joint separation because his injury apparently involved damage to muscle attachments and ligaments in his shoulder and was likely quite painful. Galen's trainer believed he had suffered a dislocation of the humerus, which could be fixed by pulling down on his arm and pushing the head of the humerus back into its correct position. Galen placed a hand in the armpit of his injured shoulder and realized there was nothing wrong with the humerus, so he told his trainer to stop pushing on the arm because it hurt and would not fix the problem.

Galen concluded that the proper treatment for his injured collarbone was immobilization although today such an injury would probably be treated with surgery.[52] He placed a tight wrapping on the injured shoulder and endured severe pain for weeks while it healed. Every day, Galen had his servants pour warm oil on his shoulder and collect it in a bowl at his feet while he kept the shoulder immobilized. The pain lasted forty days while the joint healed, and it knit so well no one believed he had ever been injured. As his reputation grew, Galen was eventually invited to serve as a physician to the emperor.

Marcus Aurelius

Marcus Aurelius was a famous Roman emperor and Stoic philosopher who lived a frugal lifestyle at a time when most wealthy Romans lived lives of hedonic excess. Modern historians respect his Stoic life, but Roman citizens disliked the limits Aurelius placed on gladiatorial games and other public celebrations. Aurelius spent much of his reign fighting Rome's enemies in northern and central Europe, especially the Germanic tribes.[53] His health was never robust because Aurelius suffered digestive and chest pains. In his treatise *On Prognosis*, Galen reported he cured Marcus Aurelius of his digestive difficulties, and the emperor was impressed. Shortly after curing the emperor, Galen left Rome for Pergamum and spent the next two years revising medical manuscripts. In AD 168, he received a message from the emperor recalling him to Rome because Aurelius was planning a military campaign against the German tribes and wanted Galen to accompany him. It's not clear whether Galen was going to serve as the emperor's personal physician or treat wounded soldiers, but he had mixed feelings about the trip and was reluctant to go with the emperor because the northern country was primitive, cold, and barbaric. However, he had no choice but to return to Rome as ordered.

Galen encountered a plague on his way to Rome although he did not say what it was. He described its symptoms, and modern physicians believe the plague was most likely smallpox. Galen reported that victims developed ulcers over their entire body, had a cough, and had scabs on their skin. He treated the disease with vinegar and mustard and applied drying medications to heal ulcers on the victims' skin. In spite of his treatments, many plague victims died, and the disease recurred periodically for years after the initial outbreak. Historians estimate that around 25 percent of the Roman Empire's population perished in this plague, which is consistent with the epidemic being smallpox because the disease is highly contagious and had a mortality rate of around 30 percent prior to the discovery of vaccines by Edward Jenner. Galen attributed transmission of the plague to breathing bad air, and smallpox can spread through atomized droplets produced by sick persons when they cough. We don't know why Galen didn't catch the disease because he was in close contact with many infected patients while treating them. Perhaps he had contracted a mild case of a similar disease (swinepox or cowpox) when dissecting animals and was immune to smallpox.[54] When he arrived in Rome, Galen was able to convince the emperor not to take him on his military campaign to the German province although we don't know how he did that.

Galen was unusually productive during the seven years between AD 169 and 176 while Aurelius was campaigning against the German tribes. He was given responsibility for the health of Commodus, the emperor's son. One afternoon, while returning from wrestling, Commodus developed a fever and asked for Galen to examine him. He took Commodus's pulse, diagnosed inflamed tonsils, and attributed the inflammation to the honey and sumac a chamberlain had prescribed. Galen ordered the honey and sumac stopped and told servants to bathe the boy when his fever subsided in two days. They did and he recovered. In AD 176, Marcus Aurelius returned to Rome for a year before going back to the German province to finish his conquest of the Germanic tribes.

Treating the Emperor

While in Rome, Aurelius developed a fever, stomach pain, gas, and diarrhea. The physicians who had accompanied the emperor in the German province recommended he rest and eat porridge. Galen was summoned to attend Aurelius and ordered to sleep in the palace for the next few days to treat him.

At first, Galen refused to take the emperor's pulse because he didn't know the character of the emperor's normal pulse and feared he would make a mistake. The emperor insisted, so Galen made his best estimate of what the emperor's pulse should be under normal circumstances and took his pulse. Galen concluded that the emperor didn't have a fever, but a digestive upset. Diagnosing a trivial digestive upset while other attending physicians suspected he suffered from a life-threatening illness was a serious risk to Galen's reputation. However, he was correct, and the emperor recovered. Galen prescribed warm ointment and peppered wine because he suspected the emperor's digestive upset had been caused by theriac, which was an antidote that emperors, senators, and other important Roman citizens routinely imbibed when they feared being poisoned by rivals. Theriac was believed to be an effective antidote to most poisons.[55]

Theriac

Theriac was taken daily by important individuals who worried they might be poisoned by rivals. The drug was originally developed to treat snake bites but was taken daily as an antidote for poison if an individual feared assassination, which most emperors did. Galen wrote a treatise *On Antidotes*, in which he listed his recipe for theriac. It contained sixty-four ingredients, including wine, herbs, honey, and the venom and flesh of live vipers. The royal palace employed a snake hunter to collect vipers so physicians could have live vipers to use in preparing fresh theriac for the emperor. Galen's recipe also contained generous amounts of opium, which had been available in the Mediterranean area since Neolithic times. Theriac was the cure-all medicine of the ancient world, probably because it contained large amounts of opium and relieved pain. The antidote was not abandoned by European physicians until the early eighteenth century.

When Emperor Marcus Aurelius died in AD 177 and his son Commodus succeeded to the throne, Galen felt anxious and uncertain about his position as a physician because the new emperor was narcissistic and emotionally unstable. However, Galen survived his time as a physician to Commodus and treated every Roman emperor until his own death in AD

216. Galen wrote extensively, conducted anatomical research, and took time to see private patients throughout his life; it's astonishing how busy Galen must have been. His diagnostic skills were renowned, especially concerning taking a patient's pulse.

The Pulse

Galen trained himself to notice small changes in a patient's pulse and often made accurate diagnoses based on that symptom alone. He studied the size, speed, strength, frequency, fullness, regularity, and rhythm of a patient's pulse to diagnose anxiety, internal growths, and fever (most often malaria). Galen believed the pulse was an accurate gauge of fever and used it extensively when diagnosing illnesses.[56] He found a tumor in one patient by evaluating the person's pulse and confirmed the diagnosis by palpating the patient's abdomen. Galen kept detailed records of the normal pulse and temperature of his patients as they aged because he wanted to compare the patient's pulse when he or she was sick with records of a normal pulse when the patient was healthy. He used differences in the patient's normal and sick pulse to diagnose various diseases.

Galen also examined urine, feces, sweat, vomit, pus, and blood from sick patients for color, texture, viscosity, and sediment to help him make diagnoses. He also noted skin color and hydration but didn't use a standard diagnostic routine when examining a patient. Instead, Galen diagnosed each patient based on the particular symptoms exhibited. He began every diagnosis by taking a complete physical and mental history, believing that past experiences and illnesses were a necessary part of any examination and that prior events could be important in reaching a correct decision about what was wrong. He recorded the patient's travels, character, temperament, and excess exertions that might contribute to an illness.

One of Galen's patients was a twenty-five-year-old man who enjoyed strenuous exercise and was industrious. The patient received bad news while on a trip and returned to his home, exerting himself on a hot and dusty journey and getting little sleep. When he arrived home, the traveler received good news, so he went to the gymnasium to exercise. While exercising, he had a quarrel with another man, broke up a fight among his friends, became dehydrated, drank water, and began to feel ill. Later in the day, the man vomited. When Galen began treating the young man, he asked him to describe his symptoms, which included recurring episodes of fever. Modern physicians would likely diagnose that Galen's patient suffered from malaria, caused by a parasite with a life cycle of forty-eight hours, which triggers recurring bouts of chills and fever. Galen did not record the diagnosis for this young patient, but if it was malaria, there was little he could have done to cure him. Perhaps Galen prescribed bleeding because it was a standard treatment at the time although modern physicians believe the procedure was actually harmful to many old or sick patients.

Bleeding

Galen took blood from patients but was careful not to withdraw too much. He believed bleeding was not helpful if a patient was weak, young, old, pregnant, or if the weather was hot and dry. However, he did not reject taking blood from patients to effect a cure, and bleeding probably contributed to some of his patients' suffering and death.[57] Modern physicians are not certain why bleeding was so popular in ancient times because there is little evidence it had any positive effect on health and may have contributed to some patients' deaths. For example, modern physicians believe George Washington's doctors may have killed him by withdrawing over 40 percent of his blood in an effort to cure him of a sore throat.[58] In addition to physical diseases, Galen diagnosed and treated mental illnesses in his busy medical practice.

Galen treated mental disorders ranging from psychoses to depression, coma, and loss of memory among his patients. He believed psychoses were caused by inflammation of the brain or the accumulation of excess yellow or black bile in the blood. Galen noted that psychoses distort reason and perception and believed that imbalances in the four humors cause most mental illnesses. He paid close attention to the mental symptoms of patients, including insomnia, delusions, anxiety, and depression. We know little about Galen's beliefs concerning mental illness because all his manuscripts were lost when the center of Rome burned in a great fire.

Fire of AD 192

The Roman fire of AD 192 occurred when Galen was around sixty-two years of age. Library and archive buildings in the center of Rome burned, destroying Galen's manuscripts and the most extensive collection of scrolls in the ancient world outside Alexandria.[59] Galen stored his important documents, pharmacological recipes, and valuable personal treasures in a room near the Temple of Peace because he believed it was fireproof. However, the doors to the building were wood; they caught fire, and the contents of the building burned. He endured plagues, famine, loss of his father, the death of his friend Boethus, and the loss of many slaves from the plague; but the fire of AD 192 caused Galen such severe grief that he wrote a treatise about how to deal with painful loss soon after. He lost gold, silver, IOUs, medical instruments, pharmacological ingredients, and manuscripts that couldn't be replaced in the fire.

Last Years

Near the end of his life, Galen summarized his thinking in two manuscripts, *On My Own Opinions* and *On My Own Books*, where he stated his final views on innate heat, the heart, nutrition, the liver, humors, the temperaments, stages of life, the efficacy of various drugs, the anatomy and functioning of the nervous system, creation, and the soul. His purpose was to clarify ideas he had developed over a lifetime of research and experiment, and because he had lost all his manuscripts in the fire, he wanted to leave a summary of his work for future physicians. Galen lived approximately twenty-three years after the fire and died in AD 216 at the age of eighty-seven years. One legend holds that he went to Egypt to study the properties of opium and died on the way. Another myth says he traveled to the Holy Land to meet the followers of Jesus and died at sea. None of these legends can be verified, and we know little about how or where he died.

After his death, Galen became a legend throughout the ancient world, and his writings became standard medical texts for hundreds of years.[60] Galen became so famous that his works were considered sacred and could not be contradicted. When Vesalius published his text on human anatomy in the sixteenth century and claimed Galen was wrong about the human anatomy, his contemporaries were outraged and rejected his conclusions until younger physicians and medical students recognized he was correct and Galen was wrong.

Chapter 3

---- ✦ ----

HUMAN ANATOMY:
ANDREAS VESALIUS

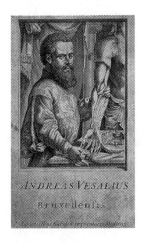

A ndreas Vesalius began dissecting human cadavers in the sixteenth century and found that Galen had made mistakes in his description of the human body because the Greek physician had based his work on animal dissections. Vesalius published an anatomy text containing two hundred beautiful illustrations of the human body that corrected many of Galen's anatomical errors. His anatomy text was criticized by the conservative medical community because it contradicted Galen's teachings, and Renaissance physicians believed that Galen was never wrong. Galen's academic career ended when Emperor Charles V appointed Vesalius physician to his household. His work in human anatomy revolutionized medical education and practice by providing physicians and surgeons with an accurate picture of human anatomy.

Andreas Vesalius was born on December 21, 1514, in Brussels, Belgium. He lived in a period of intellectual change and shifting scientific attitudes caused by the printing developed by Gutenberg in 1450, the discovery of North America by Columbus in 1492, the Protestant Reformation initiated by Martin Luther in 1517, and Magellan's circumnavigation of the world in 1519. The availability of printed books, the discovery of unknown peoples, protests against the Catholic Church, and proof the earth was round created uncertainty about accepted scientific and religious beliefs and triggered a renaissance in scientific and medical thinking.[61]

The Renaissance

European scholars began observing nature directly and thinking about man's place in the universe scientifically instead of relying on biblical teachings and church authority. The writings of Martin Luther and other Renaissance philosophers contradicted Catholic doctrine and created an upheaval among the clergy and rulers of Europe. Despite opposition from the Catholic Church, progressive philosophers and physicians found the idea of discovering knowledge through experiments appealing. The Protestant Reformation and the scientific method convinced philosophers that accepting revealed knowledge was not productive and encouraged them to study ancient medical and philosophical texts and carry out their own natural experiments. In spite of this transformation in science and medicine, conservative physicians continued to believe Galen was infallible, and his writings remained the equivalent of a medical bible that could not be contradicted by empirical observation.

The printing press made copies of rare manuscripts available at reasonable cost to medical students and the literate public for the first time. Commercial publishers could produce a thousand printed copies of an ancient Greek text for the same price as one manuscript produced by hand. Books were printed on paper rather than parchment and cost next to nothing compared to handwritten manuscripts. Moreover, printing allowed the introduction of woodcuts that produced repeatable illustrations that retained their accuracy over many printings and made ancient knowledge available to anyone who could read Latin or Greek. Printing encouraged young scientists and physicians to buy books, study ancient writings, and publish their own ideas. Vesalius was inspired by these new ideas when he began his education and became an original thinker who revolutionized the study of human anatomy.

Early Education

Vesalius was enrolled in a primary school called the Brethren of the Common Life when he was six and stayed at that institution for nine years. The school's curriculum included Latin, rhetoric, and logic. It was a Catholic school popular among wealthy Belgian families because the faculty taught accepted Christian ideas rather than critical thinking. Beginning in 1530, Vesalius studied philosophy at the University of Louvain, a well-supported college that attracted students from around the world. Just before he completed his bachelor of arts degree, Emperor Charles V declared Vesalius's father a legitimate heir to the family name, which allowed Vesalius to attend medical school at the University of Paris.[62] He traveled to Paris where Vesalius lived with Jean Sturm, a professor of dialectics and logic.

University of Paris Medical School

First-year courses at the University of Paris Medical School included pharmacy and physiology; second-year courses covered pharmacy, pathology, and surgery; third-year courses taught the origins of medicine and pathology; and fourth-year courses were reviews of physiology, surgery, and pathology. Medical students were introduced to the ideas of Galen in several of their courses and taught that his writings were infallible. That was ironic because, in his own writings, Galen advised medical students to discover the truth for themselves by observation rather than learning only from books. Vesalius read Galen and took his advice about original observation to heart. He eventually proved that Galen's works on anatomy contained errors and became world-famous as a result.

Professors at Bologna and Padua medical schools criticized Galen's anatomical works because they contained errors, but conservative medical schools continued to follow the teachings of Galen and paid no attention to claims of errors in his works made by Italian scholars. Professors at Paris Medical School believed Galen's texts were accurate and insisted their students accept his ideas as true. Dissection of a human cadaver was occasionally performed in the basement of the Hôtel-Dieu, a hospital associated with the University of Paris Medical School, but medical professors in Paris were more interested in teaching from the classical works of Galen than getting their hands dirty performing dissections. They ignored the new anatomical information being collected by dissection of the human body. Vesalius became skeptical of Galen's anatomical ideas after he began dissecting human cadavers for himself and discovered errors in Galen's writings.

Human Dissection

During the fifteenth and sixteenth centuries, knowledge about human anatomy began to change for the first time in centuries as surgeons and medical students began dissecting human cadavers. Renaissance medical scholars soon realized that ancient Greek physicians such as Hippocrates and Galen had searched for knowledge through personal observation, and they began to experiment and think for themselves.[63] Progressive physicians and surgeons developed new methods of uncovering the truth and defended their experimental procedures in the face of strenuous opposition from Catholic clergy and conservative medical colleagues. However, conservative medical professors at Paris Medical School taught Galen's anatomical works as doctrine and sought knowledge from his manuscripts rather than direct observation of human anatomy. The Paris medical faculty discouraged independent thinking and insisted students accept what Galen wrote.

The Catholic Church was strong in France, and the Paris Medical School faculty was conservative; they rejected experimentation and innovation. Even some progressive Italian medical professors attributed the errors they found in Galen's works to copying or translating mistakes rather than to Galen himself. However, Vesalius recognized that anatomy professors at Paris Medical School were more interested in translating Galen's works into Latin than dissecting human cadavers and learning the truth about human anatomy. He came to believe that personal dissection was essential to understanding anatomy, but his professors opposed the study of the human body through direct dissection. Their attitude contradicted Galen, who wrote that physicians needed to learn anatomy through their own experience rather than out of a book. Paris medical professors defended Galen's writings on anatomy without realizing his findings were based on dissections of monkeys rather than human cadavers because Roman law didn't allow him to dissect dead humans.

Professors at Paris Medical School believed dissecting a cadaver was beneath their dignity, so they delegated the task to barber-surgeons while they read from Galen's text, telling their students what they were supposed to observe during a dissection rather than encouraging them to actually observe the dissection themselves. Neither medical students nor their professors at Paris Medical School paid much attention to human dissections because they believed Galen's writings were accurate and they must not question the Greek master. However, Vesalius soon realized Galen's anatomical conclusions were inaccurate once he began dissecting human cadavers himself because Galen could only dissect animals within the Roman Empire.

Ancient Taboos

Roman, Christian, and Arab laws and beliefs forbid the study of human anatomy throughout Europe and parts of Africa in ancient times. Roman law forbade dissection of human bodies, and Christians believed the dead would be resurrected following the return of Christ, so the church demanded human bodies remain intact when they were buried, believing dissection would interfere with the resurrection of the body. In contrast, Egyptian physicians were allowed to dissect human corpses and study anatomy while they were preparing bodies for mummification. It was not until the 1300s that Italian medical professors were allowed to dissect human cadavers under strict church supervision.[64] Even then, dissections of human cadavers were performed by few physicians because it was discouraged by the Catholic Church. Not until the sixteenth century could medical students and faculty in Europe routinely dissect the bodies of convicted criminals after they were executed, and even then, human cadavers were expensive and unfit for study after a few days due to decay. Politics also interfered with medical studies in the sixteenth century because European nations were often at war, and foreign students were viewed as spies.

University of Louvain Medical School

Vesalius was forced to flee Paris during his third year at medical school because the French king rejected the authority of the Holy Roman Empire, and Charles V declared war on him. Because Vesalius was a Belgian citizen and his father was employed by the court of Charles V, French authorities considered him an enemy agent, and Vesalius had to leave France. He was disappointed to leave before finishing his studies but returned to Louvain to complete his medical education. Intellectual freedom in Belgium was not much better than in Paris, however. Vesalius found that members of the theology faculty at the University of Louvain were prosecuting William Tyndale for heresy because he had translated the New Testament into English. He was denounced as a heretic because now the Bible could be read by laymen who didn't need priests to interpret Christ's teachings. Tyndale was convicted of heresy and burned at the stake in 1536 by order of a Catholic court.

Soon after returning to Belgium, Vesalius participated in the autopsy of an eighteen-year-old noblewoman who died under mysterious circumstances. Her uncle, fearing she had been poisoned, asked for a medical examination of the body. Vesalius soon realized the barber-surgeon was incompetent, so he took over the dissection himself. After a thorough examination, Vesalius determined that the young woman had died from constriction of her thorax by a corset she wore to make her waist slim. Her uncle was grateful for his careful work and allowed Vesalius to study the young female's body in detail after the autopsy was complete.

Vesalius's return to Louvain Medical School created resentment within the faculty and admiration among fellow medical students for his skills in dissection and anatomy, so he had to tread carefully. Soon after his return, Vesalius found the body of an executed criminal outside the city gates. He smuggled the corpse into the city, cleaned the bones, and told everyone he had brought the skeleton from Paris. Vesalius kept the articulated skeleton for study and anatomical demonstrations. Vesalius presented anatomical demonstrations to his fellow medical students, effectively making him the anatomy instructor at Louvain, which created further resentment among the faculty. During one of his demonstrations, Vesalius was challenged by members of the theology faculty concerning the "seat of the soul." He refused to debate the issue, saying it was a theological, not a medical question, and he was not competent to have an opinion—an elegant tactic to avoid the controversy. Vesalius began work on his thesis so he could graduate and do research on anatomy.

Professor of Anatomy

His medical thesis, entitled *A Paraphrase of the Ninth Book of Rhazes*, was an attempt to create a comprehensive Latin nomenclature for human anatomy. Vesalius was awarded his medical degree, the thesis was published, and he was offered a position as a professor of anatomy at the University of Padua Medical School.[65] Northern Italy was controlled by the Republic of Venice at the time, and the Venetian Senate insisted that Padua Medical School hire some of its faculty from abroad. As a result, Vesalius had the opportunity to join the most prestigious medical school in the world after graduation. The University of Padua was a progressive medical school funded generously by the Republic of Venice. Its faculty members were well known for publishing scholarly texts. Vesalius was attracted to Padua because it emphasized anatomy and encouraged demonstrations of human dissection.

On December 1, 1537, he sat for a hiring examination before the dean and faculty examiners at Padua. They questioned him on all aspects of medicine and anatomy, and when the interview was finished, he was officially offered the position as professor of surgery. His teaching duties began the next day, and Vesalius performed a public anatomy demonstration. Following tradition, he dissected the abdominal cavity first, followed by the thorax, head, neck, brain, and extremities. During the demonstration, Vesalius showed those attending the demonstration illustrations he had made to clarify the lectures; the drawings contained details of the gallbladder, liver, heart, and groups of nerves with associated branches. Later, Vesalius published these illustrations in his second book titled *Anatomical Charts*. At that time, Italian art students were studying human anatomy by observing medical dissections and making sketches of the human body to improve their drawing skills. The benefits of studying human anatomy are apparent in the art of Dürer, da Vinci, and Michelangelo.

Before the Renaissance, Galen's writings were considered the best way to teach anatomy to medical students, and medical manuscripts rarely included illustrations. A text entitled *Bundle of Medical Treatise*, published in 1492, was the first medical book that included any illustrations; and *Commentary*, published in 1521, was the first anatomy book to include realistic drawings of the human body. These early anatomical illustrations were of mixed quality but helped medical students understand the structure of the human body. Vesalius believed detailed anatomical drawings were essential for teaching anatomy, and he produced a set of illustrations he planned to publish.[66]

Anatomical Sketches

Vesalius realized that realistic illustrations of human anatomy were helpful in understanding the structure of the human body, and he began using illustrations, animal dissections, and an articulated human skeleton to demonstrate features of the human body during his anatomy lectures and public dissections. His first published book contained anatomical illustrations with little text, but later he included text with the anatomical illustrations when he published his life's work. Modern medical texts make extensive use of illustrations, but they were a novelty in Vesalius's time. The appeal of Vesalius's anatomical illustrations was their large size and visual clarity; they measured nineteen inches by thirteen and one-half inches and consisted of one large drawing on a page rather than several small sketches.

He had his anatomical illustrations printed from large woodcuts so they could be held up before medical students to clarify anatomical details during his lectures. Vesalius's early anatomical drawings were intended to educate medical students about anatomy, illustrate Galen's theories of medicine, and correct a few of the errors in Galen's work that Vesalius had found through his own personal dissections of human cadavers. His illustrations were an instant success with students because they offered insights into the structure of the human body.[67] Vesalius sent a copy of his anatomical illustrations to Emperor Charles V. Other publishers, recognizing the appeal of Vesalius's illustrations, quickly plagiarized his works because there were few copyright protections in those days, intellectual property laws were rarely enforced, and books of anatomical drawings sold well.

Vesalius's early anatomical illustrations followed the outline of Galen's writings on anatomy and contained many of Galen's mistakes because he feared criticism if he corrected Galen. Later, Vesalius said he was unhappy with his first book because he knew some of his illustrations were wrong, but he published them anyway out of fear. Vesalius based later illustrations on his own observations and switched from looking to Galen's works for the truth to searching for knowledge by dissecting human cadavers and illustrating what he saw with his own eyes. In the process, Vesalius changed the content and style of how anatomy was taught to medical students by including illustrations, textural materials, and a dissected cadaver in his anatomy lessons. His revolution in medical education is followed even today.

After publishing his first book of medical illustrations, Vesalius resolved to correct the errors in Galen's texts because they were based on animal rather than human dissections. He decided to publish a complete set of revised anatomical illustrations based on his own dissections of human cadavers in the form of a medical text. Vesalius believed firsthand observation of human dissection together with an illustrated text was the best way to learn anatomy.[68] He became an expert at dissecting human cadavers by helping his anatomy teacher Guinter make detailed drawings of the human body to aid medical students in learning anatomy. Years later, Vesalius felt confident enough in his own dissecting skills, based on procedures he learned from Dutch anatomist Franciscus Sylvius, to correct Guinter's anatomy book. However, the Dutch anatomist believed Galen was infallible; and after Vesalius corrected the errors in Galen's works, Sylvius turned against him. Vesalius published his corrections to Jean Guinter d'Andernach's book in 1538, and his former teacher was not happy because the corrections suggested Vesalius was the new master of anatomy. This was not the only controversy engulfing Vesalius during his early years. He also became involved in a dispute about the best method of venesection (bloodletting).

Venesection

Venesection involves opening a small artery in the hand or foot and withdrawing blood to balance Galen's four humors. In modern medicine, bloodletting is employed to lower a patient's red cell count; but during the Renaissance, venesection was prescribed as a treatment for many illnesses. In 1539, Vesalius published a letter in which he outlined his beliefs about bloodletting. To modern readers, venesections seem barbaric; but in Vesalius's time, it was the standard treatment for correcting imbalances among Galen's four humors. One school of thought concerning venesection proposed that an artery should be cut as far from the site of infection as possible (for example, near the foot on the opposite side of the body from an infection) while the other school believed the cut to an artery should be as close as possible to the site of infection for the treatment to be effective. Based on his study of the venous system, Vesalius believed cutting close to the site of infection was the better procedure.[69] He also noted in his letter that Galen's understanding of the venous system was flawed. Vesalius based his discussion of the venous system on observations made during personal dissections of human cadavers while Galen had based his discussion of the venous system on dissections of monkeys and other animals.

Vesalius included a detailed anatomical description of human arteries and veins in his letter about venesection and shifted the search for evidence about the effectiveness of venesection from revered ancient manuscripts, such as the works of Galen, to studies of human anatomy. To oppose Vesalius's theory of venesection, a critic had to refute his direct anatomical observations rather than cite ancient Greek texts. Near the end of his letter, Vesalius said he needed to dissect additional cadavers to complete his anatomical work and reach a definitive conclusion about venesection. Modern scholars believe Vesalius's letter on venesection marks the beginning of his shift from using human dissection to support Galen's theories to investigating human anatomy and medicine independently.

After his letter on bloodletting, Vesalius began an empirical quest for truth rather than searching for evidence to support Galen. He emphasized the methodology of dissection in his book on anatomy and rejected ancient authorities as the best sources of knowledge. Later, Vesalius concluded that the study of venesection was a waste of time because it was based on a faulty understanding of veins and arteries. However, it was not until the late nineteenth century that venesection was abandoned by the medical profession.

By 1539, Vesalius was recognized as the world authority on human anatomy, and his salary was doubled by the University of Padua. In a series of innovative lectures given at the University of Bologna, Vesalius demonstrated human anatomy by combining the dissection of a cadaver with printed illustrations rather than relying solely on Galen's classical texts. He began his lecture with a summary of what he was going to demonstrate and then dissected the human cadaver, showed his students the organ in question, and explained its function and purpose. Since he had already published a treatise on the venous system, Vesalius focused these lectures on human muscles and internal organs to collect data for his forthcoming book. He also told students and physicians they should base their knowledge of anatomy on personal observation rather than on ancient texts. His students brought bodies of different ages for him to dissect; Vesalius discovered that the bones of older adults differ from young adults, and both differ from children's bones. After these lectures, Vesalius was asked to edit a Latin edition of Galen's works.

Editing Galen

In 1539, Vesalius was approached by the editor-in-chief of Giunta Press and asked to edit a Latin edition of Galen's three major works: *De nervorum* (*The Nerves*), *De venarum arteriarumque* (*The Arteries and Veins*), and *De anotomicis administrationibus* (*Anatomical Procedures*). He accepted the project with enthusiasm, believing it was an honor and an opportunity to further his anatomical work.[70] Latin was the primary language of European physicians and scholars during the Renaissance, so Vesalius planned to bring Galen's texts up to date by translating them from Greek to Latin. He also wanted to correct the errors he had found in Galen's texts. Although Vesalius was only twenty-five at the time, his goal was to publish Latin editions of Galen's works that were free of errors and reflected the latest knowledge of human anatomy based on his own observations.

Vesalius found several places where Galen's text and his own observations of human anatomy were different, so he made changes in Galen's books as he translated them into Latin. Some medical scholars accused him of blasphemy because he had changed Galen's writings. Many of Vesalius's students and friends distanced themselves as a result, and he was criticized for the rest of his life because he dared to base his books on empirical evidence rather than blindly accepting the classical interpretations of ancient texts. To counter these criticisms, Vesalius decided to publish his own anatomy book with illustrations to show Galen's errors in detail.

Fabrica

In 1540, Vesalius began to formulate his life work—an anatomy text like none before.[71] After editing a Latin edition of Galen's three famous works, Vesalius set out to find and correct all the errors in Galen's books by dissecting and observing human cadavers. He studied the anatomy of the human body through empirical dissection and based his own text entirely on observed facts rather than theoretical speculations and writings contained in ancient manuscripts. Vesalius relied on his dissections and observations to correct Galen's writings whenever he found errors. The biggest obstacle to his anatomical research was a lack of bodies to dissect. Access to bodies that were not partially decomposed was difficult, and this may explain why the sections of his text covering the skeleton and muscles were more detailed and accurate than his presentations of internal organs and tissues. By the time Vesalius reached the internal organs during a dissection, they had begun to rot and were more difficult to study than the skeleton and muscles closer to the surface.

He was also working against a publishing deadline because Vesalius had only a one-year sabbatical from the University of Padua in which to complete his anatomy text. During 1540 and 1541, he studied every one of Galen's descriptions of anatomical features and corrected them based on his own observations of human cadavers. At that time, anatomy was taught to medical students from the inside out, starting with a description of the viscera and moving out toward the extremities. Vesalius decided to present his anatomical illustrations and discussions in the same order as Galen had done in his original works. He began with the bones; progressed to muscles, arteries, and veins; covered the nervous system, the gut, the heart, and the lungs; and finally, the brain and sense organs. Vesalius included written text with his illustrations of different human organs and discussed the processes of dissection as he proceeded, giving medical students and faculty the means to test his assertions about human anatomy by dissecting a human body on their own.

His completed book contained seven hundred pages and over two hundred illustrations.[72] Vesalius wrote Latin in the style of Cicero, which made his prose difficult to read. The book was a publishing success, based more on his elegant illustrations than the detailed discussions that accompanied each drawing. Historians are not certain who drew the illustrations for *Fabrica*, but many believe the artist came from Titian's workshop. They are also not certain if Vesalius used one artist or several although the illustrations vary in quality, suggesting several artists were involved. Working with an artist was difficult because he had to be present when Vesalius performed each dissection to see the anatomical structure for himself, making scheduling the dissections more difficult. The early illustrations were better than later drawings, suggesting Vesalius was rushed toward the end and may have used several artists during the last stages to finish the book. Also, later parts occasionally relied on animal dissections and presented Galen's findings with fewer changes, suggesting that Vesalius ran out of time.

Vesalius believed that studying bones was an essential first step in understanding anatomy, so he presented the human skeleton in various poses, including one with a gravedigger's shovel under the skeleton's right arm and another showing a skeleton crying. The most famous illustrations in *Fabrica* are of human muscles displayed in layers. Vesalius presented groups of muscles and demonstrated their relationship to the skeleton in his anatomical illustrations. He showed the human body stripped of skin to display muscles in the front and side view and showed each muscle detached from the skeleton to demonstrate its anchor points on the bones.

As each sketch was completed, it was sent to the printer to be cut into a woodblock for printing. It's not known why Vesalius chose to use woodblock prints for his illustrations rather than more precise copper engravings, but perhaps it was because a woodblock could be printed on the same form (a body of type set in a chase for printing) while it was more difficult to align copperplate engravings with printed text, given the technology available at that time. Another possible reason he chose woodblocks for his illustrations was that master artisans were available in Venice to execute woodcuts. Each block carved on pear wood was expensive, but Vesalius knew that clear artistic illustrations of the human body were essential to the success of his book, and he took great care in their preparation. He even printed a special edition of his anatomy text for Emperor Charles V.

Special Edition

In the summer of 1543, Vesalius ordered a copy of his manuscript printed on vellum to create a special edition for Emperor Charles V, to whom the book was dedicated. The vellum manuscript was bound in purple velvet, with gilt edges and blue silk ties. The title page and illustrations were hand printed to make them perfect. Vesalius met the emperor personally in southern Germany near Basel, Switzerland, while Charles V was on a campaign, to present the special edition of *Fabrica*. The combination of illustrations and text in Vesalius's book created a sensation at court, in the European medical community, and among literate Europeans when it went on sale. *Fabrica* sold well because the quality and originality of the illustrations were first-rate, but the book's contents were not well received by conservative members of the medical community, who criticized Vesalius for making changes to Galen's texts.

The emperor's court physicians were shocked by the corrections Vesalius had made to Galen's texts, and conservative doctors who believed Galen was always correct resented any suggestion that their hero might be fallible.[73] Medical professors invested in teaching anatomy using Galen's texts believed their scholarship was challenged by Vesalius's publication of *Fabrica*, and they resented him. However, these conservative anatomy professors were soon rejected by their students after they studied Vesalius's book and recognized his genius and careful attention to detail. The emperor was so impressed by Vesalius's book that he made him an imperial household physician, which changed his life forever.

Before he left Italy to join the emperor's household, Vesalius was invited to present a series of anatomical dissections at the newly reopened University of Pisa. Before he arrived in Pisa, the faculty and students began collecting cadavers and bones for use in his public demonstrations. His anatomical dissections drew huge audiences, and Vesalius was asked to perform autopsies of two prominent Pisa citizens. Duke Cosimo was so impressed with Vesalius that he asked the emperor to allow the anatomist to remain at the University of Pisa, but Charles V refused. We are not certain why; but Vesalius burned his books, sketches, notes, and papers after the emperor's refusal. Years later, Vesalius said he regretted this rash act.

Imperial Physician

During his academic life, Vesalius had been able to concentrate on research and writing, but after he was appointed physician to Emperor Charles V, he was forced to leave academics though he asked several times to be allowed to return to teaching.[74] The reign of Charles V was filled with war and religious strife between Catholic and Protestant nations. As a result, Vesalius spent much of his time treating soldiers wounded in battle. Firearms had been introduced for the first time on the battlefield, and they caused wounds never before seen by physicians. Surgeons at the time believed iron or lead bullets poisoned the body, so they cauterized the bullet wounds with hot oil or a hot iron rod to counter the poison. These drastic therapies further injured the soldiers and introduced septic materials, causing infection, gangrene, amputation of limbs, and death. In the beginning, Vesalius had difficulty performing surgery on living patients because he had no experience, causing such terrible pain. He found surgery on living humans different from dissecting cadavers; the wounds were severe, and operations had to be performed quickly without anesthetics. He was clumsy at first, but after some experience, Vesalius developed several original surgical procedures for use on the battlefield.

The publication of *Fabrica* was the culmination of his life's work and the end of his academic career. His reception at Pisa reminded Vesalius he was an academic and scholar rather than a battlefield surgeon. However, because he was in the service of the emperor, Vesalius was trapped in a position he found boring and unpleasant. He hated treating common soldiers at the emperor's bidding although he made significant contributions to clinical medicine and surgery during his years of service to Emperor Charles V.[75] One of his duties was to embalm the bodies of nobles killed in battle, and this allowed him to make detailed anatomical studies although conditions on the battlefield made these studies crude and incomplete. Vesalius developed a less traumatic way of treating gunshot wounds using unguents to cover the wound and avoid infections rather than cauterizing them with hot oil or a hot iron rod.

None of the physicians and surgeons of that era understood the theory of germs; they believed infections were inherent in the wound itself rather than being caused by germs introduced on unclean instruments or dirty surgical hands. Surgeons at that time didn't understand that germs could fall directly from the air onto an open wound, causing sickness or death. While working as an army surgeon treating wounded soldiers, Vesalius was recalled to attend the emperor.

Emperor's Physician

In the spring of 1545, Vesalius was recalled from his post as an army surgeon to treat the emperor. He was met with disdain by the Spanish physicians who had been attending Charles V because they feared for their positions if this famous anatomist took over his care. Charles V suffered from asthma and other respiratory ailments all his life and developed gout as an adult due to his diet and lifestyle. Gout causes swelling of the joints because the body is unable to excrete the excessive uric acid contained in the rich food aristocrats consumed. Meats that contain large amounts of purine were especially likely to cause the production of excess uric acid and lead to gout. Charles loved fried kidney, liver, heart, sardines, and anchovies along with beer and wine at his meals. These rich foods combined with a sedentary lifestyle caused Charles serious health problems. Vesalius advised the emperor to modify his diet and exercise more to cure his gout, but the emperor refused. Because of the pain caused by his gout, Charles constantly searched for a miracle cure but never found one. Vesalius treated the emperor at his palace and opened a private medical practice among the nobles in Charles's court.

Private Medical Practice

In 1546, Vesalius established his own private medical practice and began studying clinical medicine because he believed it was a neglected field. His reputation grew as he diagnosed and healed prominent knights and the emperor himself. One of his patients suffered from severe pain in his inner right thigh that made it impossible for the knight to eat or sleep. Vesalius surgically opened the thigh where the pain was located and scraped infected pus from the wound. The knight's pain diminished soon after the surgery, and he began to eat and sleep comfortably once the incision healed. This is the first recorded case of surgery being used to treat a bacterial infection. Vesalius also surgically treated cases of empyema, a collection of pus in the pleural cavity caused by a lance or sword wound to the chest. His treatment was successful in curing many penetrating wounds in the chest cavity. Modern doctors use a similar procedure to treat chest infections by surgically inserting a tube in the chest to drain pus from an infected lung.

In 1558, Vesalius made a correct diagnosis of the illness suffered by Maximiliaan, Count of Buren, who was returning from England on a diplomatic mission. Vesalius examined the count and announced he had only a few days to live because he was suffering from an advanced abscess in his upper thorax between his lungs and announced that the infection was untreatable. After several such insightful diagnoses, Vesalius became famous for his accurate prognoses and successful treatments. Anatomical research remained the foundation of his clinical practice, giving Vesalius insight into the location and likely cause of pains and diseases. Vesalius decided to visit Jerusalem near the end of his life before he died.

Visit to the Holy Land

In 1564, Vesalius left Spain by ship for the Holy Land.[76] He stopped in Venice, and records suggest he was offered and accepted his old position as professor of anatomy at the University of Padua before leaving for Jerusalem. As he sailed across the Adriatic Sea, the ship encountered a violent storm that lasted several days. The ship ran low on food and water, and those on board began to die. The small ship finally landed in the harbor at Zante, a Greek island that was part of Venetian territory. Vesalius was seriously ill when he left the ship and died soon after. The exact cause of his death is unknown, as is the location of his tomb.

Chapter 4

---✦---

CIRCULATION: WILLIAM HARVEY

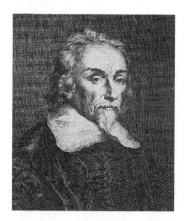

William Harvey clarified how blood circulates in the human body and introduced the experimental method to medicine. Galen believed veins originated in the liver, arteries originated in the heart, the liver produced blood that flowed back and forth in veins, and the heart worked like a bellows. Harvey showed that Galen's theory of circulation was wrong by dissecting human cadavers, performing some of the first scientific experiments on live animals, and observing blood circulating in a transparent shrimp he found living in the Thames River. He was able to observe the transparent shrimp's circulation through a magnifying glass and saw blood enter the right side of the heart via the vena cava and flow out through arteries when the heart contracted. He also observed blood flow via the pulmonary artery into the brachia (the breathing organ of shrimp)

and saw the contracting left ventricle of the heart push blood through the aorta to the rest of the body. Harvey showed that blood returns to the heart through veins that contained valves that allowed blood to flow only toward the heart.

Harvey was born on April 1, 1578, and entered King's Grammar School at the age of ten to learn Greek, Hebrew, and Latin. He enrolled in Cambridge College at age fifteen to study rhetoric, ethics, logic, music, arithmetic, astronomy, and geometry. Going to lectures was compulsory; and students were required to take verbatim notes, write essays, and defend their thesis before an audience. After graduating, he entered Cambridge Medical School.[77]

Cambridge Medical School

Harvey enrolled at Cambridge Medical School in 1598. It was not a first-class medical school, so he organized an independent course of reading with his tutor and three other medical students. Harvey did most of his studying in the library where chained texts were available for use by students. He would select a book and read while standing at a table because students could use a book for no more than one hour at a time. Harvey spent hours copying and memorizing passages from Galen so he could answer his tutor's questions. He paid special attention to Galen's theory of how the heart worked because he wanted to do research on circulation after he graduated.[78]

Galen believed there were two circulatory systems: veins originating in the liver, and arteries originating in the heart. He wrote that the liver produced blood that carried nutrients to the body through veins, that blood flowed back and forth in veins, and was drawn to the various organs by a mysterious force he didn't understand. Galen thought the heart worked like a bellows, drawing blood from the lungs and sending it to the body with each beat.

In 1599, Harvey left Cambridge because he contracted an illness. Modern experts speculate that he suffered from malaria because Harvey experienced shivering and fever, both symptoms of the disease. When he recovered, Harvey entered Padua Medical School, which attracted bright students from all over Europe because it was considered the best medical school on the continent and Harvey wanted to obtain a first-class medical education.[79]

Padua Medical School

In 1600, Padua was the intellectual center of the Venetian Republic, and its medical school offered a safe haven for Protestants such as Harvey. A few months after he entered Padua, Harvey was elected leader of the English students at the school. The faculty at Padua Medical School wanted students to have hands-on experience in medicine, so they required all medical students to accompany practicing physicians on their rounds. Students learned to diagnose illnesses, predict the course of diseases, talk to patients in a comforting manner, collect a comprehensive medical history, and prescribe treatments under the direction of practicing physicians. Poor patients were treated by inexperienced medical students and often suffered as a result. Students learned to mix medicines using plants and herbs grown in the school's botanical garden. Padua medical professors focused on the works of Aristotle rather than Galen in their teaching.

Harvey became interested in studying circulation early in his medical career, perhaps because religious doctrine taught that a man's life was recorded on his heart, and on Judgment Day, God could see whether he was righteous or evil. Galen also believed human emotions occur in the heart. For Aristotle and Galen, the heart occupied a central place among human organs because it was considered to be the seat of intelligence, emotions, and the soul. Whatever the reason, Harvey spent much of his professional life studying human circulation. But first, he had to learn human anatomy.

Learning Anatomy

Padua Medical School owned a circular dissecting theater that held two hundred fifty spectators and offered them a reasonable view of a cadaver on a table in the center of the room. The theater contained five galleries, each three feet higher than the one below. Wooden rails kept the audience from falling to the floor, and medical students were assigned to the lower galleries so they could see dissections up close.[80] Student leaders occupied front-row seats in the lowest level of the theater, and that's where Harvey sat every time a dissection occurred. Dissections were offered during December and January when it was cold and a cadaver would not decay so quickly. City officials, local aristocrats, and rich merchants were invited to sit in the lower seats to view dissections. Porters tried to maintain order during the dissections; but bored students sometimes threw objects at each other, shouted insults, and disrupted the lectures.

The anatomy theater was designed to limit noise, but it was still loud with so many people packed into one small space. When the audience was seated, the professor of anatomy would stride in and begin his lecture. The demonstration followed traditional lines, with the professor reading from a book, a barber-surgeon doing the dissecting, and an assistant pointing to various organs as the professor described them. Often, the professor ordered the dissecting to be completed ahead of time so the lecture could proceed more quickly. A century earlier, Vesalius had recommended that the professor himself carry out the dissection, describe the various organs, and point out the highlights of each organ system as he proceeded. However, anatomy professors at Padua didn't want to get their hands bloody so they hired barber-surgeons to do the cutting.

The purpose of studying anatomy and natural philosophy was to appreciate God by understanding his design of man. Professors at Padua followed the teachings of Aristotle rather than Galen and tried to define the cause (pattern or form) of each organ along with its structure and function. During a public dissection, the anatomy professor would describe the organ under review and explain its action (efficient cause) and role in maintaining life. Next, the substance (material cause) of the organ was explained to show how it performed its action (efficient cause). Then the purpose (final cause) of the organ was described. Anatomy professors at Padua examined organs in isolation rather than describing their interrelations and covered the structure and function of sense organs, reproduction, respiration, muscles, bones, and other systems in different lectures.

Once a human organ had been examined, the anatomy professor would have an animal brought in so he could demonstrate the same organ to his students for comparative purposes. The human cadavers were generally young criminals whose executions were timed to coincide with medical school dissections. Following hanging, the criminal's body was transported to the university for dissection; afterward, it was given a Christian burial by city officials. Harvey was fascinated by dissection, committed anatomy lectures to memory, and earned high marks in medical school. He began his final examination for a medical degree on April 25, 1602, before a count who had the power to award medical degrees under Venetian law. The oral examination took the form of a disputation (a formal system of debate in the Middle Ages designed to uncover the truth) in which the medical student was expected to show his mastery of medical theory, fact, and rhetoric through discussion and questioning. Harvey easily passed the examination and was presented with a medical insignia (a snake curled around a shaft), a gold ring, a doctor's cap, and books on philosophy and medicine.[81]

His father was present when Harvey received his medical degree and must have been delighted to see his son become a doctor. Harvey planned to open his own medical practice in London the following year after taking time off to visit his family.

London Physician

In 1602, after spending a few months with his family, Harvey opened his medical office near St. Paul's Cathedral in London. Two years after he established his practice, Harvey married Elizabeth Browne, the well-connected daughter of prominent London physician Lancelot Browne, on November 24, 1604.[82] His father-in-law was a fellow of St. John's College, Cambridge; a member of the College of Physicians in London; and the royal physician to King James. Thomas Harvey gave his son a house in London as a wedding present, and his father-in-law facilitated Harvey's appointment as physician to the Tower of London, vouching for his learning, honesty, loyalty, and discretion. Lancelot Browne also helped Harvey become a member of the College of Physicians in London, an institution established by Henry VIII to supervise the practice of medicine in London. The College of Physicians granted licenses to London doctors and prosecuted persons who practiced medicine without a license.

In England, doctors enjoyed high status compared with barber-surgeons and apothecaries. They wore purple gowns, were addressed as "master," and were able to charge high fees. Because London was plagued by smallpox, tuberculosis, and other endemic diseases, there were ample patients available for trained physicians to treat. On May 4, 1603, Harvey presented himself before examiners from the College of Physicians to obtain a license to practice medicine in London. He was examined in Latin and asked to define an element, epilepsy, colic, and ague. When the examination was finished, Harvey received permission to practice in London and was told he would need to undergo three more examinations before gaining formal licensure as a physician.

Harvey rose quickly within the College of Physicians, becoming censor, treasurer, and one of the members eligible to elect the next college president. He prosecuted untrained persons who claimed to be doctors and inspected apothecary shops to determine if their medicines were pure and prepared according to the standard formula. Harvey appeared before the King's Privy Council to lobby for stricter laws and higher fines for shops that adulterated medicines and asked Parliament to require barber-surgeons to have a physician attend their operations. The barber-surgeons fought back, arguing that physicians were only interested in collecting fees because their presence at operations was unnecessary. The London citizens who had little faith in physicians or surgeons attempted to cure themselves by appealing to God or one of the saints rather than seeing a doctor and paying his fee.

Harvey's younger brother was a footman in the king's service and gave him an entrée to the royal court. He acquired manners appropriate for the court of King James and learned how to deal with titled ladies and gentlemen. Harvey wore the right clothes, danced, gossiped, and flattered the court aristocrats. He eventually became the royal physician to King James, who was a difficult patient because he was sensitive to pain. After James died in 1625 from a stroke and dysentery, his son Charles appointed

Harvey physician in ordinary, an important post that carried an annual salary of three hundred pounds. Harvey's duties included treating the royal household and accompanying them on trips around the English countryside. He also became chief physician of a large London hospital.

Hospital Physician

On February 25, 1609, Harvey applied for the post of hospital physician at St. Bartholomew's Hospital in London.[83] He was recommended by the king, so the hospital governors approved his appointment quickly. Six months after he joined the hospital, the chief physician died, and Harvey was promoted to fill the position. St. Bartholomew was one of two large London hospitals where Catholic sisters nursed sick patients. As chief physician, Harvey consulted with the hospital staff and surgeons once a week in the Great Hall where he also treated patients. He would examine each patient, diagnose their illness, prescribe medicines, and give advice. Harvey was courteous, listened to their complaints, took their pulse, and examined their urine before making a diagnosis.

The hospital apothecary mixed the medicines Harvey prescribed and dispensed them to each patient according to the chief physician's directions. Harvey treated over four hundred hospital patients annually with medication, surgery if required, better food, and comfortable living conditions. He examined patients every week and decided if they were able to leave or needed further care. His private practice prospered even though jealous London physicians accused Harvey of malpractice, which was common in that competitive medical community. He treated mostly noble families and rich merchants who were able to pay his fees. Harvey became an important London physician and decided to apply for a coat of arms to confirm his social status.

Coat of Arms

Harvey accumulated a fortune through his lucrative private practice, his position as chief physician at St. Bartholomew's Hospital, and his appointment as physician to the royal family. He sued patients who didn't pay, lived frugally, ate simply, invested in real estate, and lent money at interest. Around 1614, Harvey applied to the king for a personal coat of arms, a privilege generally granted only to men of noble birth. To qualify, Harvey had to show he possessed a fortune of several hundred pounds, dressed well, kept servants, and had funds to bribe the right officials. Highborn gentlemen complained that ordinary Englishmen could gain a title by paying money rather than through a family pedigree, but the king needed funds and encouraged the practice. Harvey was granted his coat of arms, and his father died in 1623 knowing his son was a certified gentleman.

In 1615, the College of Physicians appointed Harvey a lecturer in anatomy, offering him a generous stipend and the prestige of representing the college. He lectured in English to barber-surgeons because they did not understand Latin. Barber-surgeons had begun as assistants to monks who treated poor patients but could not perform the surgery themselves because of their religious beliefs. Later, barber-surgeons began assisting physicians and medical school professors during operations and public dissections. During his lectures to the barber-surgeons, Harvey dissected one body to show the muscle systems, another to demonstrate the skeleton, and a third to explain the thorax, abdomen, and sense organs because corpses decayed quickly. Dissection of the viscera was most difficult because it took time to expose these internal organs and they deteriorated quickly. Most dissections were performed during cold winter months to slow decay, but rotting was still a problem. Harvey discussed the function and purpose of each organ as he proceeded through his lectures.

In addition to anatomy lessons, Harvey offered a course on surgery and dissection to the barber-surgeons. He followed the dissecting style of Vesalius, making incisions himself, explaining what he was doing, pointing to and describing the structure and function of each organ as he proceeded. Harvey used candles to illuminate the organs he was dissecting so students could see inside the body, and he wore a white hat and apron with detachable sleeves he could change when they became bloody. Harvey paid particular attention to dissecting the heart and circulatory system because he wanted to understand how they worked.

The Heart

Before discussing the structure and purpose of the heart, Harvey removed the breastbone and ribs, cleaned fat from around the heart, and used a candle to show his students the exposed human heart. He explained that the heart was dense thick flesh, compact, and hot because it was filled with blood. Harvey pointed out the vena cava, which collected blood from veins and delivered it to the right side of the heart and traced the arteries from the heart through the thorax into the neck and head. He made an incision in the right side of the heart to expose the inside of the vena cava and inserted a rod to show how it sent blood to the lungs. Harvey also showed how the pulmonary artery carried blood to the lungs. He next made an incision in the left ventricle of the heart and pointed out how it sent blood to the rest of the body.

Early in his career, Harvey taught the conventional theory of circulation according to Galen, being reluctant to present his own ideas when they contradicted the Greek master's teachings. He explained the differences he found between Galen's description of human anatomy and the body he was dissecting by suggesting that the human body had changed since Galen's time rather than suggesting that Galen might have been wrong. Harvey taught Galen's theory that blood circulated by ebbing and flowing through arteries and veins and that the liver manufactured blood, which was consumed by the organs. Galen believed the heart's active phase occurred when it expanded, drawing blood through the veins, but Harvey eventually discovered that Galen's theory was wrong and developed a new model of circulation that revolutionized medical thinking about how the heart functions.

During later anatomy lectures, Harvey explained how Galen

believed circulation worked and then discussed an alternate theory of circulation, which assumed blood was forcefully ejected from the heart when it contracted. Harvey's alternate theory of circulation assumed that the systole phase (when the heart contracted) moved blood through the arteries, contrary to Galen's theory that it was the diastole phase (when the heart expanded) that moved blood through veins.[84] Harvey described his own observations of the heart and said he believed Galen might have been mistaken about exactly how the heart worked. At the conclusion of the anatomy lecture, Harvey took questions from his audience, and several older physicians criticized his comments contradicting Galen's theory of circulation because they believed Galen was infallible. At the end of each demonstration, Harvey examined the body on the dissecting table to decide if it could be used for another lecture. If the body showed too much decay, a new corpse would be brought in and prepared for the next day's dissection. In addition to lecturing and treating patients, Harvey carried out research on human circulation during evenings in his private laboratory.

Private Research

Between 1610 and 1620, Harvey was exceptionally busy with his work at St. Bartholomew's Hospital, his private practice, attending the royal family, and lecturing on anatomy. In spite of his busy schedule, each evening, he returned home, had dinner with his wife, changed into work clothes, and went to his private laboratory to conduct research on human circulation. His laboratory contained a dissecting table, instruments, anatomy books, and a menagerie of living animals, including toads, crabs, geese, rabbits, mice, sheep, pigs, and dogs. Harvey's goal was to develop a description of every organ in the human body and explain how it functioned. He intended to compare human and animal anatomy and develop an understanding of the structure, function, and purpose of human organs. Above all, Harvey wanted to understand human circulation and determine if Galen was correct about how the human heart functions.[85]

Harvey wanted to study the differences he discovered between Galen's theories and his own observations and understand how blood circulates through the heart and around the body. He collected executed criminals' bodies and brought them to his private laboratory to dissect. Harvey opened their chests to expose the heart, blood vessels, and lungs for study. In his first experiment, Harvey inserted a small tube into the right ventricle of the heart and injected water under pressure, causing the right ventricle to swell. He noted that no water flowed from the right to the left ventricle of the heart, contrary to Galen's description of human circulation. In this one simple experiment, Harvey demonstrated that Galen's theory was wrong, but he still needed to discover the true nature of circulation for himself and experimentally demonstrate how the heart worked. Harvey knew he would need strong evidence to prove Galen was wrong because most physicians believed Galen was infallible and would not easily accept criticism of their hero.

Harvey injected water into the right ventricle in his second experiment and found it flowed out through the pulmonary artery and back to the left atrium (left upper chamber of the heart). This result suggested to Harvey that blood was oxygenated when it passed from the right ventricle of the heart through the lungs and then flowed back to the left atrium of the heart. Harvey decided he needed to perform a systematic set of experiments to show how blood circulates during the heart's active and passive phases before he shared his theory with others. He decided to begin dissecting living animals so he could actually see blood flowing through a living animal, but found that their heartbeats were so rapid he was unable to observe what actually happened when contraction and expansion of the heart occurred. He did notice that when his animals began to die, the heart beat slower and he could observe circulation for a short time before the heart stopped beating.

By observing the slowly beating heart of a dying animal, Harvey concluded that contraction of the heart constitutes its active phase as blood is sent from the heart through arteries to various organs. But he still didn't have a clear picture of how blood circulates throughout the human body. He needed to study living animals to understand circulation in detail, and he didn't know how to do that because the normal heart rate of the animals he was studying was too rapid and, when they were near death, he only had a short time to observe the heart's function before it stopped. Then Harvey had a critical insight—he decided to study cold-blooded animals, whose metabolism was slower than the warm-blooded animals he had been using.[86]

Cold-Blooded Animals

Harvey stopped dissecting warm-blooded animals such as dogs and began dissecting cold-blooded animals such as frogs and fish. He found that the hearts of cold-blooded animals beat more slowly at low temperatures than the hearts of warm-blooded animals, so the function of a living heart was easier to observe. Harvey studied several cold-blooded animals before he discovered a shrimp living in the Thames River that had a transparent body that enabled him to see its heart beating through a magnifying glass without having to do any dissecting. He noted that blood flowed through the shrimp's arteries when the heart contracted and became convinced Galen was wrong about how human circulation occurs.[87]

Harvey then cut open a living cod and observed its heart beating and put his finger on the heart to feel the muscle. He noted that when the heart contracted, it became hard. Since he knew voluntary muscles become hard when they move limbs, he had solid evidence that contraction was the active phase of the heart, which sent blood through arteries to the lungs and body. Harvey then cut open an eel and observed that the eel's heart became white and hard when it contracted. He was convinced the heart was a muscle, and when it contracted, the heart expelled blood into arteries.

Experiments on Circulation

Harvey returned to dissecting warm-blooded animals to confirm the ideas he had developed in observing frogs, fish, shrimp, and eels. He placed a living dog on the dissecting table, tied it down, and exposed its beating heart. Harvey had to work carefully to avoid killing the animal before he could collect useful information about its circulation. He observed that blood entered the right side of the heart via the atrium, and when the heart contracted, blood was driven from the right ventricle via the pulmonary artery into the lungs. At the same time, the contracting left ventricle pushed blood out through the aorta to the rest of the body. To test his theory, Harvey tied off the dog's right vena cava and saw that the pulmonary artery collapsed because it was receiving no blood. Meanwhile, the left ventricle of the heart continued to force blood through the aorta to the body. Harvey then loosened the tie on the vena cava and saw blood rush back into the empty right ventricle of the heart and out through the pulmonary artery to the lungs. He was getting close to understanding how human circulation works.

Harvey noted that arteries expanded when the heart contracted, suggesting contractions were causing the human pulse. He tested this idea by tying off the aorta of a dog, observed that the pulse stopped beyond the ligation, and resumed when he released the tie. Harvey concluded that the pulse represents the propulsion of blood through arteries when the heart contracts. Next, he sliced an artery while the dog's heart was beating and saw blood spurt from the artery in time with each heartbeat. When the animal died, the heart stopped beating, and the blood stopped spurting from the cut artery. Harvey was astonished by the amount of blood spurting from the artery when it was cut because Galen had claimed that blood was produced in the liver and consumed by the organs, muscles, and tissues. If Harvey's observation of the amount of blood flowing from the severed artery was correct, the liver would have to produce much more blood than seemed physically possible. He estimated that over six thousand ounces of blood were pumped by the average human heart in a day. Harvey didn't believe the liver was capable of manufacturing that amount of blood every day. He also wondered why the body didn't become flooded with fluid if that amount of blood was created daily. Harvey believed he understood how circulation worked in animals and, by analogy, within the human body, but how could he be certain that animal and human circulation were identical without examining a living human heart? And how could he do that ethically? Harvey got lucky when he was referred a patient who had suffered an unusual wound in his chest as a child.[88]

Studying a Living Human Heart

Harvey examined a young nobleman who, as a child, fell, broke a rib, and injured his chest. The chest wound became infected, a large amount of pus drained out of the wound, and when the child recovered, he had a gap in his chest that showed the movement of his internal organs through the opening. When Harvey examined the young nobleman, he realized he was seeing a beating human heart through the gap in the nobleman's chest. Harvey could actually observe a beating human heart and study circulation in a living human. He cleaned the gap in the man's chest and brought him to the king for examination. Harvey and the king each placed a finger on the nobleman's heart and concluded it was insensitive to touch. Harvey asked the king to observe the beating of the heart and tell him whether blood was expelled from the heart when it contracted. The king observed the heart and agreed that blood flowed from the heart when it contracted. Harvey now had proof in a living human being that blood was expelled from the heart when it contracted.

He believed blood must return to the heart so it could be pumped out again rather than being consumed by the various organs, but he didn't understand how that occurred. He believed arteries carried blood from the heart to the lungs and body, but where did the blood go after it was pumped through arteries to the organs, and how could it return to the heart to be recirculated?

Veins

Harvey knew blood was transported to organs through the arteries because when he tied a cord around a patient's arm, the arteries above the cord swelled while no blood flowed through arteries below the cord. When he released the cord, Harvey saw the arm regain its color as blood flowed through arteries to the hand. It was obvious to him that blood was carried to the hands and feet through the arteries, but what happened after that? He speculated that blood flowed back to the heart through veins and decided to find out through a simple experiment. Harvey recalled a demonstration he had seen at Padua Medical School when one of his professors exerted pressure on a vein in an attempt to force blood through it toward the hand but found that it was impossible. Harvey speculated that there must be little valves in veins that allow blood to flow from the hands and feet toward the heart but block blood from flowing back through the veins toward the hands and feet. Harvey confirmed this speculation by dissecting a vein above and below a valve and showing that blood could not flow away from the heart toward the extremities in a vein no matter how much pressure he exerted.[89] He concluded that little valves in veins were one-way gates that allowed blood to flow toward the heart but not toward the feet or hands. Harvey now believed he understood how blood circulates throughout the human body.

Harvey's Theory of Circulation

Harvey thought blood is propelled by heart contractions through arteries, and returns to the heart through veins, encouraged on its way back to the heart by valves in veins that allow blood to flow only toward the heart. He also believed blood is infused with air in the lungs, sent to the left auricle of the heart, and expelled by the left ventricle through arteries to the body before returning through veins. Harvey could not actually see how blood was transferred from arteries through organs to veins at that time because microscopes were too crude to allow him to actually view tiny capillaries, but he speculated that very small arteries (capillaries) must transfer oxygenated blood to an organ, and very small veins (capillaries) must collect the blood from the organs and return it to the heart. Even though he could not see these capillaries, Harvey believed blood flows to the body through arteries and back to the heart through veins in a continuous loop. He also believed blood follows a double path: one through the lungs from arteries to veins and another through the body from the heart through arteries to organs and back to the heart through veins.[90] His theory contradicted the work of Galen and was going to cause Harvey endless troubles over the next few years as he presented his findings to the medical community.

Criticism of Harvey

Between 1618 and 1628, Harvey demonstrated his theory of circulation to numerous groups, including the king. He invited members of the College of Physicians to watch a demonstration of circulation in his private laboratory. Harvey told his audience he would explain and demonstrate his theory concerning the function of the heart and the circulation of blood through the human body. He said blood passes from the right ventricle of the heart to the lungs through arteries and from the lungs through veins back to the left ventricle of the heart, from which it is expelled to the body through arteries by contractions of the heart, flows through organs, and back into veins before returning to the heart. He concluded that blood is driven through arteries by contractions of the heart, passes through the organs, and returns to the heart through veins that have one-way valves that allow blood to flow only toward the heart.

Harvey announced to the audience that he intended to prove these statements by presenting various demonstrations so his listeners could evaluate his theory for themselves. He showed that the septum (the separation between the right and left ventricles of the heart) is impervious by forcing water into the heart and noting that it didn't flow directly from one ventricle to the other. He also demonstrated the flow of blood through the pulmonary artery to the lungs, the expulsion of blood by contraction of the left ventricle through arteries to the body, the function of small valves in veins that allowed blood to flow only toward the heart, the pulse of blood through an artery when the heart contracted, and the circular movement of blood through arteries and veins. During these demonstrations, Harvey dissected several animals and made arguments to support his theory. When he finished, the fellows of the college attacked his theory because it was contrary to Galen's ideas.[91] One fellow asked if a large amount of blood spurting from the cut artery might not be the result of the wound itself rather than the beating of the heart. Another asked if the heart of an eel is really comparable to the heart of a man. Members of the College of Physicians offered numerous irrelevant objections because they were committed to believing Galen and wanted Harvey to be wrong.

Galen taught that four humors reside in separate areas of the body, and imbalances among these humors cause illnesses. If Harvey's theory of blood circulation was correct, Galen's four humors would mix automatically as blood circulated throughout the body, and Galen's theory of humors could not be correct. According to Galen, the heart balanced and regulated humors, but did not mix them. Harvey expected criticism because his theory contradicted Galen's teachings and called into question basic therapeutic techniques such as bloodletting, but he expected intelligent physicians to at least consider his evidence. He was wrong; older conservative colleagues refused to believe Galen might be in error and wouldn't even consider Harvey's evidence supporting this theory of circulation.

Harvey also understood that if the heart mixed blood in a healthy individual, bloodletting was unlikely to fix imbalances of the four humors and was probably a useless medical treatment. His attempts to deal with these criticisms through experimental evidence didn't convince conservative physicians who were committed to believing Galen and, as a result, rejected Harvey's evidence as irrelevant. They simply couldn't accept Harvey's evidence because it contradicted the theories of Galen.[92] He was unable to convince members of the College of Physicians that his theory of circulation was correct because their minds were closed. They stuck with Galen and criticized Harvey's ideas in spite of clear evidence supporting the new theory. Surprised but not discouraged, Harvey decided he would publish his research and allow the medical community to reach the right conclusion on its own in good time.

Publication

In 1628, Harvey published the results of his research on circulation in a book titled *De motu cordis*.[93] He began with a description of how he discovered that forceful contractions of the heart caused the human pulse. Next, he described a large amount of blood forced into arteries when the heart contracted. Then he explained how blood is circulated to the lungs through arteries, back to the heart through veins, and how blood follows a circular path from the heart through arteries to organs and back through veins to the heart. Harvey presented each argument in a single chapter, along with critics' objections and his responses to their criticisms. He edited the book several times before making a final copy of the manuscript and sending it to Frankfurt for publication by William Fitzer. Unfortunately, the printed book contained a few errors, either because of Harvey's poor penmanship or negligence by the publisher.

Older members of the College of Physicians continued to insist they didn't agree with Harvey's theory of circulation, but medical students and younger physicians praised his work, and professors of anatomy concluded that Harvey's theory of blood circulation was elegant and correct. Despite hostility from the older medical community, a majority of young physicians in England and Europe accepted Harvey's theory of circulation after he published his book. When he became famous, other physicians began claiming they had discovered the correct theory of circulation before him although none could point to any published evidence to support their claims while supporters of Galen continued to attack Harvey's theory at every opportunity. Meanwhile, England was about to enter a bloody civil war that would have serious consequences for Harvey.

English Civil War

The conflict began when King Charles called Parliament into session to pass a tax so he could pay off accumulated debts. Parliament refused to pass the tax until the king renounced his claim to be "above the law." Charles rejected Parliament's demand, and relations between the monarch and Parliament settled into a hostile standoff. In 1642, the English Civil War erupted when the Roundheads marched against King Charles and his Royalist Army.[94] Harvey stayed loyal to the king and continued to treat the royal family and wounded noblemen during the war. After six years of war, the Royalists were defeated, King Charles beheaded, and the English Commonwealth established under the leadership of Oliver Cromwell. Harvey was in serious trouble by this time.

Harvey's Last Years

Cromwell announced that Harvey was a delinquent because he had supported King Charles during the Civil War and confined him to London. Harvey's wife died from natural causes, and his medical practice failed after the war because noble patients could no longer afford his fees. He suffered serious pain during his last years and even asked a physician to help him die, but the friend refused. Ironically, Harvey bequeathed his fortune to the College of Physicians to build a museum and library named after him. At the official opening of the building, Harvey was elected president of the college. Seventy-nine-year-old Harvey suffered a stroke and died on June 3, 1657.[95]

Chapter 5

---------- ✦ ----------

ANIMALCULES: ANTONIE VAN LEEUWENHOEK

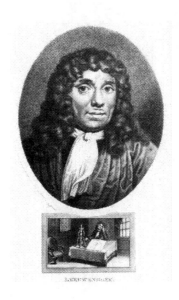

Antonie van Leeuwenhoek developed lenses that could magnify objects five hundred times and was curious about everything in nature. He collected water from lakes and other sources to study under his microscope and was surprised to see tiny creatures he called "animalcules" swimming in the samples. They looked like tiny snakes, were smaller than a strand of hair, and came in various colors. He described his observations in a letter to the Royal Society that included detailed drawings of the small creatures he saw. The Royal Society was skeptical of his claims and asked Robert Hooke, their expert on microscopic lenses, to investigate Leeuwenhoek's findings. Hooke was unable to see the small animals Leeuwenhoek had described until he manufactured a better magnifying lens. When Hooke reported his conclusions to the Royal Society, they were impressed by Leeuwenhoek's discovery and made him a member of the society. Leeuwenhoek also verified Harvey's theory of circulation by observing blood flowing from arteries through tiny capillaries in an organ and back through tiny capillaries to veins, confirming by microscopic observation the circuit Harvey thought must exist, but could not see.

Leeuwenhoek was born on October 24, 1632, in Delft, the Netherlands. Before he was six, two sisters and his father had died, leaving his mother with five young children to raise. She remarried and Antonie was sent to a boarding school in Warmond where he learned to read and write. Later, Leeuwenhoek lived with his uncle in a small village north of Delft where he learned reading, mathematics, and science. When he was sixteen, Leeuwenhoek's stepfather died, and his mother sent him to Amsterdam to work in a linendraper's shop to learn the trade. One of his jobs was to examine fabrics with a hand lens to determine their quality, and that experience triggered Leeuwenhoek's lifelong interest in magnifying lenses. After six years at the linendraper's shop, he returned to Delft to open his own drapery shop and marry his childhood sweetheart, Barbara de Mey, in July 1654.[96]

Leeuwenhoek spent evenings after work reading about the natural world and using his magnifying lenses to study small objects, including his skin, the hairs on his hand, the wood grain in a table, and other small items. He discovered that things look different through a magnifying lens compared with regular vision, and he began making drawings of what he saw. In addition to managing his drapery shop and reading about nature, Leeuwenhoek participated in city affairs and increased his income by becoming chamberlain for the Delft sheriff. Leeuwenhoek worked as a chamberlain for over forty years and experienced serious personal losses.[97]

Personal Tragedy

Leeuwenhoek's mother, one of his sisters, and his wife died, leaving him a widower at thirty-four with a ten-year-old daughter. Five years after his wife died, Leeuwenhoek married Cornelia Swalmius, whose father was a minister. His second marriage gave Leeuwenhoek the opportunity to discuss his microscopic studies with his father and brother-in-law, both educated men who read Latin and could understand what he was doing. In 1669, Leeuwenhoek became a land surveyor and was placed in charge of wine imports in Delft, increasing his income further. By the time he was forty, Leeuwenhoek had accumulated significant savings, his surviving child was grown, and both his wives had died, so he decided to close his shop and devote himself to making better magnifying lenses and studying the microscopic world. In the process, he pioneered the field of microbiology and became a famous amateur scientist.

Leeuwenhoek studied bacteria from his mouth, the vacuole of cells (the small space within a cell enclosed by a membrane), human spermatozoa, and muscle fibers (muscles are composed of single-fiber cells banded together and move the body). He also collected samples of water from various sources, such as watering troughs, wells, lakes, and seawater. In these samples, Leeuwenhoek found small creatures swimming in the liquid when he looked through his magnifying lens. He saw creatures that scientists call germs, which are single-celled animals that live in the air, water, soil, and the bodies of animals and plants. He also manufactured better magnifying lenses so he could see smaller and smaller creatures.

Magnifying Lenses

Historians don't know a great deal about his scientific activities between 1660 and 1673 because Leeuwenhoek stopped keeping a personal journal during those years or they have been lost. Perhaps he became secretive because he was experimenting with making better lenses at that time so he could see smaller things, and that may explain the absence of personal journals. Leeuwenhoek was dissatisfied with the magnifying lenses available at the time because they had two major faults: spherical and chromatic aberration.[98] Spherical aberration means straight lines at the edge of a field of view appear curved when viewed through an uncorrected magnifying lens, and chromatic aberration means that the edges of objects appear to be blurred and colored blue or yellow, interfering with seeing the magnified image clearly.

These aberrations were worse in a compound microscope (which uses two lenses to magnify an object) compared with a single-lens microscope. The most famous lens maker in the world at that time was Robert Hooke, curator of experiments at the Royal Society, who wrote a book about the microscope in 1665. Hooke said he didn't use single-lens microscopes although they made objects clearer and could magnify as much as a compound microscope (he called it a double microscope) because using a single-lens microscope strained his eyes. Hooke said that if an observer could tolerate the eyestrain, a single-lens magnifying glass was superior because its chromatic and spherical aberrations were smaller and would disturb vision less compared with a compound microscope. Historians don't know if Leeuwenhoek was aware of Hooke's book, but he spent years learning how to make better magnifying lenses so he could view smaller and smaller objects and make detailed drawings of them. Leeuwenhoek didn't invent the microscope, however.

Invention of the Microscope

Galileo Galilei is credited with inventing the first single-lens microscope in 1609, and Dutch spectacle maker Zacharias Janssen is believed to have discovered the principle of constructing a compound (double lens) microscope at around the same time.[99] The compound microscope works by placing a lens at each end of a metal tube and passing light through the tube, creating a magnified image that can be seen through the eyepiece. One lens focuses and enlarges a beam of light from the surface or through the object to be viewed while the other lens increases the magnification of the object. Magnification in a compound microscope is the sum of the objective and eyepiece lens magnifications, allowing the compound microscope to produce a larger image than is generally possible using a single magnifying lens. However, Leeuwenhoek was able to craft a high-quality lens that magnified objects nearly five hundred times, which was extraordinary at the time. He used his superior lenses to make single-lens microscopes for his own use.

Leeuwenhoek's Microscopes

Leeuwenhoek created more than five hundred lenses during his lifetime, and eight of them have survived to the present day. His best surviving microscope magnifies more than 275 times, but historians believe he must have produced lenses that had the power to magnify an object nearly 500 times to have seen some of the small creatures he sketched in his notebooks.[100] His microscopes were housed in a frame made of copper or silver that held one of his specially made lenses. His single-lens microscope measured about five centimeters on each side (about two inches), and he held it near his eye and looked toward the sun to produce adequate light for viewing magnified objects. On the opposite side of the lens from Leeuwenhoek's eye was a pin or a glass slide on which he attached or placed the material he wanted to observe.

Leeuwenhoek added three screws to the back of his microscope to make it easy to use. One screw focused the object he was viewing by moving it closer or farther away from the lens, and the other two screws moved the object he was viewing in two dimensions so he could observe its different parts. He mounted solid specimens on the end of a pin or glued them to a small rod mounted behind his magnifying lens to hold them in place while he made his observations. Leeuwenhoek looked at fluid specimens in a pipette he manufactured or smeared the fluid between two thin plates of glass to make a slide so he could see and record his observations. Leeuwenhoek never revealed how he made his high-quality lenses, so historians are not certain what process he used. In 1957, C. L. Strong created similar lenses by using thin glass threads he manufactured by heating and stretching a glass rod, which he snapped into two parts. Strong then heated the end of each thin glass rod to create a round glass lens. Based on Strong's work, historians believe Leeuwenhoek probably created his lenses by a similar process of heating a glass rod, pulling it into a thin glass thread, breaking the thread, and heating the end of the glass thread to create a round lens capable of magnifying objects.

Leeuwenhoek kept his lens-making technique secret so he could make discoveries and publish them before anyone else. When he examined these new lenses, Leeuwenhoek found they increased the size of an image many times more than existing lenses. He not only made excellent lenses, but Leeuwenhoek was also a first-class observer who made the most of his new lenses. His special skill at using a magnifying lens led Leeuwenhoek to make a major discovery—the samples of lake water he collected and observed under his microscope contained small living creatures no one had ever seen before.[101]

Berkelse Mere

Leeuwenhoek was experimenting with glass pipettes to improve the clarity of liquids he was studying and decided to collect and look at water from Berkelse Mere, an inland lake about two hours from Delft. The lake water was reported to be clear in the winter, but turn whitish with little green clouds floating in it during the summer. Local villagers believed the water changed color because of dew falling into it, but Leeuwenhoek wanted to learn for himself what was causing the color change. He collected samples of the lake water during the summer and placed them under his microscope to see what was causing the color change. He placed a pipette full of lake water under his microscope, lifted it to his eye, and he could not believe what he saw. Leeuwenhoek observed several different tiny creatures swimming around in the lake water. He called them "animalcules."

Leeuwenhoek said they formed spirals similar to the copper spirals distillers use to cool liquors during distillation. He also reported that the creatures were smaller than a grain of sand or a strand of hair and were alive and moving about. Leeuwenhoek may have been observing green algae or protozoa, which have round or oblong shapes. Other creatures he observed in the lake water had two small legs near their head and two fins at the end of their bodies. These may have been rotifers. Other small creatures were elongated and moved slowly. Perhaps they were ciliates. The animalcules he observed came in different colors, including white, transparent, or green in the middle and banded in white.[102] Other tiny creatures he saw were gray or green. Leeuwenhoek wrote that many of the creatures moved rapidly in the water and were several times smaller than anything he had seen before.

He wondered what these small creatures could be and whether they were unique to the waters of Berkelse Mere or could be found elsewhere in samples of water. He was thinking like a trained scientist and asking interesting questions. Leeuwenhoek studied the lake water at different times of the year to see if the creatures were there all the time or only during certain times in summer and found that they were more numerous during the summer. He also decided to collect and study other samples of water to see if animalcules were widespread or unique to the Berkelse Mere. He discovered that small animals similar to those in the lake water were present in most water samples he collected.

Leeuwenhoek also looked at human hair, the brain of a fly, a moth's wing, and a piece of dust, among other objects. He studied various microorganisms found in different samples and made drawings of a broad range of biological specimens using his superior lenses. Leeuwenhoek had no idea what he was observing but believed he had stumbled on something important.[103] No one had ever seen these small creatures before, and he wanted to understand their habits and distribution before reporting his findings. Leeuwenhoek didn't realize the images he was seeing with his new lenses would produce two new branches of science: protozoology and microbiology. A friend convinced Leeuwenhoek to send a letter to the Royal Society with detailed drawings of the small creatures and other objects he was studying to get their reaction to his discovery.

The Royal Society

One of his neighbors, Dr. Regnier de Graaf, brought Leeuwenhoek a copy of *The Philosophical Transactions*, the official publication of the Royal Society of London, and told him that there was an article in it about an Italian who had made a microscope and observed a small animal with it. De Graff asked if he could contact the Royal Society and tell them about what Leeuwenhoek was doing and seeing. Leeuwenhoek was not intimidated by the Royal Society, so he said "yes" to de Graaf. His neighbor sent a letter to the Royal Society, along with a letter from Leeuwenhoek describing his microscope and including drawings of the small creatures he had seen. Members of the Royal Society were skeptical when they first received Leeuwenhoek's letter of October 6, 1676, illustrating the very small organisms he had observed. In the letter, he described creatures he saw in lake water, the stinger and mouth of a bee, and a louse. No one had ever seen such small creatures before, and members of the Royal Society doubted they existed.

In response to their skepticism, Leeuwenhoek affirmed that he had seen the single-cell creatures he had drawn and sent the Royal Society letters from prominent Delft citizens verifying they had also seen the same small creatures in Leeuwenhoek's microscope. Still skeptical, the Royal Society asked Leeuwenhoek to send them one of his microscopes so they could replicate his work, but he refused because he didn't want anyone to see how he had manufactured his lenses. After his refusal, the Royal Society asked their curator of experiments, Robert Hooke, to repeat Leeuwenhoek's experiments and see if they were true.

Replication of Leeuwenhoek's Work

Hooke tried, using the magnifying lenses he had available, but could see nothing in the lake water samples he collected.[104] Hooke was convinced Leeuwenhoek and the Delft citizens who sent testimonials about his work had seen the small creatures Leuwenhoek described in his microscope, but he was unable to see the same creatures with the lenses he had on hand. He decided to make a better lens and thinner pipette before he rejected Leeuwenhoek's claims. After manufacturing several better magnifying lenses, Hooke was finally successful in seeing the small creatures Leeuwenhoek had drawn. He showed his results to the assembled Fellows of the Royal Society, and they were impressed with Leeuwenhoek's claims now that Hooke had verified them.

In the meantime, Leeuwenhoek invited the Royal Society to send a delegation to his home in Delft to look through his microscope and verify that they could actually see these small organisms for themselves. However, members of the Royal Society said that was not necessary because Robert Hooke had verified the observations and they believed him. Leeuwenhoek's claim that he saw single-cell organisms was accepted, his letter was translated into Latin, published, and he was made a member of the Royal Society, a singular honor for an uneducated man. The Royal Society invited Leeuwenhoek to send additional reports with more drawings of what he observed, and he sent regular letters describing his studies to the Royal Society for his entire life.

Letters to the Royal Society

In his second letter, Leeuwenhoek reported that he had little formal education but would try to describe the observations he was making in as clear a way as he could. The Royal Society became even more interested in Leeuwenhoek's work after Sir Constantijn Huygens, Dutch diplomat and father of scientist Christiaan Huygens, wrote to the Royal Society and told them Leeuwenhoek was a most curious and industrious man and recommended they take him seriously. *The Philosophical Transactions*, the official publication of the Royal Society, collected and published letters from all over Europe, acting as a clearinghouse for new scientific ideas. Contributors ranged from professionally trained scientists, physicians, architects, and linguists to gifted amateurs such as Leeuwenhoek. The fellows of the Royal Society met weekly and suggested interesting research topics for others to pursue. Their suggested research ideas included the growth and use of potatoes, the history of cloth dying, forest development, weather studies, how to make a clock, and experiments on gravity.

Leeuwenhoek continued to make new discoveries almost every time he looked at a new sample of water or other material. In another letter to the Royal Society, Leeuwenhoek reported he had seen what is now called *infusoria*, a word describing small aquatic creatures such as ciliates, euglenoids, protozoa, single-cell algae, and small invertebrates that exist in freshwater ponds. Leeuwenhoek had found these little organisms in a drop of pond water. These microorganisms are assigned to the kingdom Protista and are used to feed newly hatched fish.[105] Infusoria can be cultured by soaking organic matter in a jar of fresh water for a few days and can be detected by the naked eye as small specks moving around in the jar of water held up to sunlight. However, what's visible with the unaided eye is sunlight reflecting off small creatures in the water. To see the creatures themselves requires a microscope. Leeuwenhoek was fascinated with small organisms and collected them from various sources for study.

Dental Bacteria

He observed small creatures in tartar scrapings from his own teeth. Based on descriptions of his observations, Leeuwenhoek was likely seeing bacteria although he didn't know about germs at the time. It would be almost two centuries before the germ theory of disease was established experimentally by Robert Koch. Generally, the little creatures Leeuwenhoek collected from his teeth were alive, but one day, he found they were all dead. To learn why Leeuwenhoek stopped cleaning his teeth for three days and then scraped tartar from them to study under his microscope. He found many small organisms in these scrapings from his teeth when the tartar was mixed with water. Next, he rinsed his mouth with wine vinegar and took more scrapings. Now Leeuwenhoek found only a few small organisms still living in the tartar taken from his teeth after rinsing with vinegar while he had seen many creatures in the scrapings taken before he rinsed with vinegar. Next, he mixed wine vinegar with the tartar and water, studied it under the microscope, and saw the small creatures die within minutes. He concluded that vinegar was killing the small organisms in his mouth. Later, Leeuwenhoek studied soft tissue from one of his decayed teeth.

Leeuwenhoek had no idea there was a connection between the bacteria he was observing in his mouth and tooth decay. He had taken the tartar from healthy teeth in his mouth and collected samples of tartar from other healthy persons, not realizing these tiny creatures he was observing could damage teeth over time. He did speculate that the small creatures he was observing might be the cause of bad breath. Leeuwenhoek developed decay in one of his teeth, and the crown broke off. He collected soft matter from the root of his decayed tooth, mixed it with water, and studied the preparation under his microscope. Leeuwenhoek saw thousands of small creatures swimming around in the soft matter extracted from his decayed tooth, but he didn't realize these bacteria might be causing the tooth decay. Earlier, Christiaan Huygens had suggested there might be a connection between the small creatures Leeuwenhoek was seeing in his magnifying glass and disease, but too little was known at that time to substantiate such a theory. Two centuries later, Louis Pasteur showed that yeast is involved in wine fermentation and that bacteria cause the wine to sour, laying the foundation for germ theory that was later developed by Robert Koch. Leeuwenhoek studied a wide range of subjects with his microscope, including small insects.

He studied the life cycles of various insects; described the eyes, brain, and feet of a housefly; and found that fleas are attacked by mites. Leeuwenhoek described seeing basketlike hairs on the legs of a bee, which he believed were used for carrying pollen from plants back to the hive. He studied the bee's mouth, eyes, and stinger, but couldn't find a nose anywhere. Biologists now know that bees breathe through tiny holes on each side of their bodies and don't have a nose. Leeuwenhoek reported that the horns of a louse have five, not four joints, as claimed by Robert Hooke, and he noted the common louse was active and difficult to observe. He tried cutting off its head, but the louse continued to move for some time after it was decapitated.

Leeuwenhoek lived during a period of rapid scientific progress that was often opposed by the Catholic Church.

Science and the Church

After the printing press was invented, science expanded rapidly due to the availability of books that allowed more individuals to read about the latest scientific advances. The scientific method produced new ways of thinking about the world, and scientists came to believe that truth could be discovered by observation and logical thinking rather than only coming from revelations or teachings of the Catholic Church.[106] However, these radical new scientific ideas drew opposition from the clergy. In many Catholic countries, especially Italy, scientific ideas were suppressed by the Roman Catholic Church. For example, the church criticized the findings of Galileo Galilei, who suggested that experimental observations with scientific instruments such as the microscope and telescope could generate new theories of how the world originated and functioned. Church leaders saw these radical ideas as a threat to their authority, excommunicated Galileo, and forced him to recant his theories. Rene Descartes, another natural philosopher, argued that education should train students to think for themselves and use mathematical methods to study nature rather than simply learning accepted religious doctrines, and the church opposed his teachings as well.

In spite of opposition from the church, more and more educated men came to believe that scientific study could yield progress and make life better for all mankind. Leeuwenhoek was free to continue his work and publish his observations without censorship, including his studies of human blood, because the Netherlands was Protestant and tolerated scientific thinking.

Studies of Blood

Leeuwenhoek was curious about everything, including the structure of blood and how it circulates. We are not certain what aroused his curiosity; perhaps he cut his finger and decided to see what blood looked like under his microscope. In any case, Leeuwenhoek began a systematic study of blood by collecting a sample in a small pipette or smearing some on a glass slide, mounting the sample behind his lens, and systematically observing his own blood through the microscope. Leeuwenhoek reported that he saw small round globules floating in clear liquid when he viewed human blood.[107] He noted that when blood was exposed to air, it became brighter in color before coagulating. At first, he believed blood corpuscles were round, but later realized they were flat ovals. He estimated that a blood cell was around two hundred forty times smaller than a grain of sand. Not content to study his own blood, Leeuwenhoek collected and studied blood from various animals, including cod and salmon, which contained little red oval blood cells. He also studied how blood circulated in various animals, including rabbits, bats, and fish.

Leeuwenhoek knew nothing of William Harvey's earlier work on how blood circulates in the human body when he began studying blood circulation in a rabbit's ear, a bat's wing, and a small fish under his microscope. Harvey deduced the basics of human blood circulation through ingenious experiments but was unable to observe how blood moved from arteries through organs and back through veins to the heart. He couldn't see the small capillaries within organs because Harvey didn't have the excellent lenses Leeuwenhoek manufactured. Leeuwenhoek verified Harvey's speculation about circulation by directly observing blood flowing from arteries through capillaries within various organs and returning through veins to the heart, confirmed by microscopic observation the circuit Harvey assumed must exist. Leeuwenhoek also noted that when an animal's heart contracted, blood flow increased through the small capillaries he was watching. In addition to manufacturing excellent lenses, Leeuwenhoek developed several original scientific procedures for studying small creatures in a microscope.

Scientific Methods

Not only did Leeuwenhoek produce superior microscopes, but he also developed systematic procedures for observing and recording what he saw and asked basic questions about the small creatures he was studying. He distinguished between fact and speculation, kept detailed records of his observations in a manner similar to Leonardo da Vinci, and tested his theories with further study and observations rather than accepting his initial speculations as facts. Leeuwenhoek made drawings of what he saw through his lenses so others could verify his work. These drawings are so accurate that hundreds of years later, scientists can often identify the small creatures he was seeing. Leeuwenhoek also helped develop the branch of science concerned with studying small plants and animals by slicing and staining them for observation under a microscope.[108]

Histology

He learned how to slice cross-sections of plants thin enough so he could study their cellular structure under a microscope. Leeuwenhoek was one of the first to study the structure of opaque objects by cutting them into thin slices, staining them with dyes, and viewing the resulting specimens through his microscope. He made thin slices of cork and parings from a quill pen by using a sharp razor and found he could see the material's structure if he held the slice of material toward the sun under his microscope so that bright sunlight passed through the thin translucent material, allowing him to see its structure in detail. Leeuwenhoek studied the structure of coffee beans in 1687 by roasting the beans in an oven, cutting them into thin slices, and looking at the soft interior of a bean under his microscope. He noted that when the bean slice was pressed before he placed it under his microscope, Leeuwenhoek could see oil in the sliced coffee bean. Leeuwenhoek was the first to stain microscope specimens with saffron so he could differentiate the structure of an object in better detail.[109] The Royal Society published almost two hundred letters from Leeuwenhoek, and they attracted the attention of kings and emperors.

Royal Interest

After he was admitted as a Fellow of the Royal Society, Mary II of England, wife of William III, stadtholder of the Netherlands, visited Leeuwenhoek's home in Delft, hoping to see his microscopes for herself. He was absent when she arrived because he was on vacation, but when Leeuwenhoek learned of her visit, he sent Mary two of his better microscopes so she could see animalcules for herself. Mary was delighted with the gift and showed the microscopes to members of the English court. Dr. Thomas Molyneux, physician, biologist, and official representative of the Royal Society, visited Delft where he examined a dozen of Leeuwenhoek's best microscopes. The doctor wanted to purchase some of the microscopes to take back to London for use by the Royal Society, but he was told they were not for sale. In 1698, Leeuwenhoek was visited by two representatives of Czar Peter the Great of Russia, who asked him to meet on a ship anchored south of Delft in the harbor. Czar Peter wanted to see his microscopes and have Leeuwenhoek explain what he was doing. Leeuwenhoek was honored and immediately set off to visit the ship. The Russian welcomed Leeuwenhoek in fluent Dutch and asked to see his microscopes.[110] Peter had come to the Netherlands to learn about Dutch shipbuilding and worked in the Dutch shipyards himself to learn how they constructed their excellent sailing ships. Leeuwenhoek was so pleased with Peter's interest in his work that he gave the emperor two of his better microscopes to take with him to Russia.

Near the end of the seventeenth century, Leeuwenhoek had a virtual monopoly on the microscopic study of small zoological creatures because his lenses were superior to any others available at the time. He studied many different small organisms and tried to estimate the number of them in various samples of water. Leeuwenhoek described one small creature that consisted of four or five clear globules without skin or outside membrane. He noted that when these small creatures moved, they stuck out two little horns that were in continuous motion. He described other small creatures that had round bodies and tails nearly four times as long as their bodies. Modern scientists believe he was describing a species of vorticella, often found attached to submerged objects at the bottom of harbors. Leeuwenhoek speculated that they moved by stretching out and pulling in their tail but later realized the creatures were not swimming with their tail, but attaching themselves to underwater objects with it.

He described another animalcule that had an oval-shaped body and many little legs that moved. When he removed these creatures from the water, they formed a round shape, swelled up, and burst. Modern scientists believe he was observing and describing protozoa, which are small creatures with no skeleton or skin. Leeuwenhoek had no idea that his discoveries would make him famous when he began making lenses and looking at small things in his microscope. He studied these small creatures out of curiosity because he wanted to find out what was in the water and liked to look at things through his microscope. Leeuwenhoek studied many small things to see what they looked like through his microscope. His curiosity ranged from studying samples of lake water to investigating the hot taste of pepper.

Studies of Pepper

One day, Leeuwenhoek began wondering what caused the hot taste of pepper and decided to find out. He speculated that the hot taste of pepper was caused by little needles that trigger pain on the tongue.[111] To test his theory, he tried tasting pepper that had been soaked in vinegar for a year. Finding that the vinegar-soaked pepper tasted hot on his tongue, Leeuwenhoek set out to discover what caused the sensation. He took peppercorns, ground them into a fine powder, mixed the powder with water, and waited for several days, adding water to the mixture as the liquid evaporated. After three weeks, he examined the water with his microscope and found that there were four kinds of animalcules swimming in the pepper infusion. Three were similar to small creatures he had seen before, but the fourth was so small he said it would take one hundred of these creatures in a line to be the size of a sand grain.

Leeuwenhoek tried another experiment in which he took well water that contained many different small creatures and added some coarsely ground pepper. He observed the water one hour later and noted that the small creatures had slowed their motion. After twelve hours, only a few of the creatures were still alive; after two days, all were dead. A few days later, Leeuwenhoek saw new animalcules moving in the pepper water. One was a new large round specimen he had not seen before. In a few more days, Leeuwenhoek observed more small creatures swimming in the ground-pepper water, including little eels, lying together and wiggling. He wondered if a jar of vinegar he had stored in his basement also contained small creatures, so he placed a sample under his microscope. When he first observed a sample of the vinegar from his cellar, he saw nothing.

But after eleven days, he observed small eels in the vinegar, and their number increased over time. He added pepper to the vinegar and found the little eels died. Leeuwenhoek concluded that pepper was killing the small creatures, but he still hadn't discovered what caused pepper's hot taste. Today, scientists know the hot taste of pepper is caused by capsaicin, an oily chemical that binds with sensory neurons on the tongue to make a person believe he or she is experiencing heat on the tongue. Leeuwenhoek also wanted to understand the origin of life, so he studied the theory of spontaneous generation.

Spontaneous Generation

Leeuwenhoek was a meticulous observer who designed experiments that produced repeatable results. He was willing to trust his own observations and argue against accepted scientific doctrines if his experiments suggested the theory was wrong. He became interested in testing the theory of spontaneous generation, which proposed that life developed spontaneously from inorganic matter and not just from other life through cell division or sexual reproduction. Leeuwenhoek knew that the small microorganisms he had observed divided or reproduced more of themselves rather than developing spontaneously from the filth in water, and he believed these observations contradicted the theory of spontaneous generation, which was an early explanation for the origin of life. Leeuwenhoek often saw small animals divide while he was observing them through his microscope, suggesting to him that new life formed from other life and not from spontaneous generation.[112]

He was an experimental scientist who changed his mind based on his own observations, and he concluded that life doesn't develop spontaneously, but only comes from other living things through cell division or reproduction. To prove that living things come only from other living things and that all organisms have parents, Leeuwenhoek asked people to send him grains of wheat that contained weevils. He combined the wheat containing weevils with pest-free wheat he has stored for some time in a sealed container and separated the mixture of wheat and weevils into three glass jars. In a fourth jar, he placed weevils without any wheat. He discarded the fourth sample in twelve days because all the weevils had died from lack of food. Leeuwenhoek observed weevils in the three jars that contained wheat and noticed that the small animals hollowed out the wheat over time.

After two weeks, he observed that the weevils in his three jars with wheat grains were coupling, with the female carrying the male around piggyback fashion. A few days later, he observed small maggots among the weevils and wheat. Leeuwenhoek examined grains of wheat from each of the three jars containing weevils under his microscope and found eggs, maggots, and weevils of varying sizes. He concluded that weevils deposited their eggs on the outside of a grain of wheat, and when a maggot hatched from the egg, it bored into the grain of wheat for food. He believed that weevils only grew from eggs laid by pregnant females and didn't appear spontaneously from inorganic matter. Not content to base his conclusion on the study of just one species, Leeuwenhoek studied a grain moth as well to see if it could spontaneously produce new life from dead creatures. He placed eight grain moths in a glass jar, added a little sulfur to the jar, lit it with a match, and watched the moths die from the sulfur fumes. He waited several days and noticed that the dead moths produced no new offspring. He studied other creatures as well, such as ants, flies, and fleas to see if they developed spontaneously from dead parents. None did. Leeuwenhoek concluded that life comes only from life through reproduction or producing live offspring by cell division rather than from spontaneous generation from inorganic matter. This was one of his last major microscopic studies as he grew older.

Last Years

In 1716, when Leeuwenhoek was eighty-four years old, the University of Louvain awarded him an engraved silver medal in appreciation of his lifetime of work. The silver medal was sponsored by the professors of medicine and philosophy at the University of Louvain to commemorate his discoveries in natural philosophy. During his last years, Leeuwenhoek sent letters to the Royal Society describing weakness in his hands and legs and dimness in his right eye. He wrote what he believed was his "last" letter to the Royal Society, but Leeuwenhoek lived another five years. He died at the age of ninety on August 26, 1723, and was buried within the Oude Kerk in Delft.[113] Most of his microscopes were sold by his family after his death, and many were lost over the ensuing centuries. Eight are known to have survived, and five of his original microscopes are held in a museum in the Netherlands.

Chapter 6

---- ✟ ----

VACCINATION: EDWARD JENNER

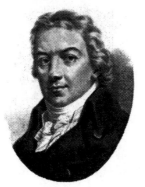

Edward Jenner.

E dward Jenner studied cowpox for years trying to understand how to transfer this mild disease from infected to healthy children and give them immunity to smallpox. He collected and published fifteen case studies of persons who had contracted cowpox naturally and another nine cases of children Jenner intentionally infected with cowpox to prove that natural infection or artificial inoculation with cowpox protected children against smallpox. However, Jenner's cowpox inoculations didn't always create immunity to smallpox, and he wondered why. He found that serum taken from a pustule between the fifth and eighth days after a child produced cowpox symptoms produced the most effective vaccine for inoculating children against smallpox, and heating cowpox serum or storing it for several days caused the serum to not work. Prior to vaccines, up to 80 percent of children who contracted smallpox and more than 400,000 Europeans died each year. Jenner's discovery of vaccination saved millions of lives and contributed to a huge increase in population that began in England during the eighteenth century.

Edward Jenner was born May 17, 1749, in Berkeley, England. His father enrolled him in Wotton-under-Edge Grammar School when Jenner was eight. Due to an outbreak of smallpox in the area, Jenner was variolated by a local physician, which meant he was infected with variola minor, the less severe form of smallpox.[114] Variola minor has a mortality rate of approximately 2 percent while variola major, the severe strain of smallpox, has a mortality rate of around 30 percent among unvaccinated children. Because physicians at that time believed it was inevitable that children would contract smallpox, many were intentionally infected with variola minor smallpox in the hope they would survive this relatively mild form of the disease and be immune to variola major, the real killer of children.

Jenner survived the variolation and moved to Cirencester when he was nine to study the classics and language with Reverend Dr. Washbourn. He found studying the classics dull, so Jenner apprenticed with John Ludlow to become a surgeon.[115] Little is known of the years Jenner spent as an apprentice learning medicine and surgery, except that when he finished, he was well qualified to practice medicine. An examination was required before a doctor could practice surgery in London, but none was needed when Jenner opened his practice in the country. He apparently obtained a good medical education working with Ludlow, watching him treat patients, and studying medical texts because his colleagues were impressed with Jenner's knowledge and skills. After he finished his medical apprenticeship, Jenner was hired to classify plant specimens collected by Joseph Banks, a botanist who accompanied Captain Cook on his round-the-world voyage between 1772 and 1775. Banks was so impressed with Jenner's work that he helped him become a member of the Royal Society.[116]

Since he had inherited land from his family, which gave him ample income from rents, Jenner decided to do medical research rather than concentrate on his practice. He contacted John Hunter, a surgeon and medical researcher in London, and they collaborated on several projects. Jenner also became socially active in his community, wearing the latest London fashions, developing good manners, and acquiring modest musical skills so he was welcomed into the better homes in his area. In 1788, he married Catherine Kingscote.[117] It was a fine marriage for Jenner because Catherine had an ancient family pedigree and a well-connected physician father. Jenner was thirty-nine, and Catherine twenty-seven when they married. Soon after, his mentor and friend John Hunter died of a heart attack following an argument with a member of a medical committee. Jenner was saddened by his death but was not surprised because Jenner had noticed signs of heart disease in his colleague for years. Jenner began looking for a new research topic following Hunter's death and became interested in the idea of vaccinating children against smallpox after listening to a paper presented at his local medical society.

Cowpox Vaccination

On July 18, 1789, Jenner's friend Dr. Henry Hicks presented a lecture on swinepox in which he reported that the disease seemed to confer some immunity to smallpox.[118] Shortly after Jenner heard the paper, swinepox was diagnosed in a young girl who had been a nurse for Jenner's son, and he decided to test the theory that cowpox could create immunity to smallpox in children by taking serum from a swinepox pustule on the infected girl and inoculating his son and two other young children. A modern ethics panel would be shocked by this experiment on children with no earlier animal studies, but it was not an unusual practice in Jenner's day because the death rate from smallpox variolation was around 2 percent and swinepox or cowpox inoculation was believed to be much safer than variolation with smallpox minor. The children developed a few pustules around the inoculation sites after nine days but experienced no serious symptoms. Weeks later, Jenner variolated the children with variola minor smallpox, but they developed no smallpox pustules, indicating the inoculation had immunized them against smallpox. Jenner decided to study how cowpox created immunity to smallpox by collecting additional data, hoping future physicians could avoid inoculating children with variola minor and risking death.[119]

Modern physicians know that cowpox, monkeypox, and smallpox are all members of the orthopox family of viruses, and if a person is infected with any orthopox virus, he or she will be immune to that entire viral family, including strains of smallpox.[120] The fact that any member of the orthopox family of viruses will inoculate individuals against smallpox was confusing to Jenner and his contemporaries, and that uncertainty produced arguments over the proper way to vaccinate against smallpox. Physicians at that time didn't understand how vaccination worked or what the proper method of extracting and storing serum from cowpox pustules was to preserve its effectiveness, so Jenner needed to learn how to inoculate children effectively with cowpox serum. Sometime between 1791 and 1793, Jenner wrote a note to the local Medico-Convivial Society, saying he had observed that individuals who were naturally infected with swinepox or cowpox were immune to smallpox and he intended to study the process in detail and develop a procedure to inoculate children against smallpox. This is the first publication suggesting children could safely be vaccinated against smallpox by using serum from cowpox rather than by inoculation with variola minor smallpox, the mild form of smallpox, which had a death rate of 2 percent.

Jenner studied cowpox inoculation for years, trying to understand how to vaccinate children effectively against smallpox.[121] At first, he distinguished between "true" cowpox and "spurious" cowpox to explain why some children he inoculated with cowpox later contracted smallpox. Later, he learned that the more likely reason some of his early cowpox inoculations were ineffective was because he hadn't collected the cowpox serum at the proper time from a patient and did not know how to store the serum to preserve its effectiveness. Another problem for Jenner was that cowpox disappeared from cattle herds for unknown reasons, only to reappear a year or two later, so he sometimes had no animal source of cowpox serum for inoculation. Also, he didn't understand how to store the serum properly to preserve its effectiveness.

To avoid having to rely on cowpox from cattle when he was gathering evidence for the theory that cowpox inoculation gave children immunity from smallpox, Jenner decided to transfer cowpox directly from an infected child to a healthy child rather than from cattle to children. He wanted to prove it was possible to transfer cowpox from one human to another, and he was not concerned that infecting children with cowpox posed an ethical problem because variolation against smallpox had been done by physicians for years, and vaccination with cowpox posed little risk because it was not lethal.[122] Symptoms of cowpox infection can include pustules on the skin, swelling in the armpits, a fever, joint pains, headache, and low energy, but not death. In contrast, vaccination with variola minor causes death in about 2 percent of unvaccinated children, and contracting smallpox major results in death approximately 30 percent of the time among unvaccinated children.

Case Studies

The first donor of the cowpox serum Jenner used in his experiment transferring the disease from one child to another was a young woman named Sarah Nelmes, daughter of a farmer near Berkeley parish. Sarah contracted cowpox through a thorn scratch while milking cows, a fairly common occurrence among farm children. Jenner collected serum from Sarah's skin and infected a healthy boy of eight named James Phipps with cowpox. He made two small incisions in the boy's arm, dipped a clean lancet in the serum from one of Sarah's cowpox pustules, and placed the serum in the incisions he had made on the boy's arm.[123] Four days later, redness appeared around the incisions; and five days after that, two pustules formed at the site where Jenner had placed the cowpox serum. James Phipps experienced a mild fever and low energy for a few days and recovered.

After his recovery, Phipps was variolated with smallpox minor on July 1, 1796, to determine if the cowpox inoculation was effective against smallpox. Jenner waited fourteen days, the known incubation period of smallpox, before he was certain the boy was immune because he developed no smallpox symptoms after variolation. Jenner had performed the first successful cowpox inoculation by taking cowpox serum from Sarah and transferring it to James. After this single success, Jenner was convinced that inoculation with cowpox could prevent smallpox infections, and he decided to publish his preliminary result in the *Transactions of the Royal Society*. He submitted a short paper to the society in October 1796, describing his experiment with cowpox vaccination on James Phipps. However, the Society decided not to publish his work because it "appeared too much at variance with established knowledge." Jenner decided he needed to collect more cases to support his inoculation theory before resubmitting his paper.[124]

Additional Evidence

Jenner collected two types of cases for his expanded paper: fifteen cases of children who had contracted cowpox naturally and another nine cases in which Jenner intentionally infected each child with cowpox. He tested the children's immunity to smallpox by variolation.[125] Case 1, Joseph Merret, caught cowpox from an animal, was variolated and found to be immune to smallpox. Case 2, Sarah Porlock, contracted cowpox naturally and resisted infection with cowpox serum at a later date. Case 3, John Phillips, had contracted cowpox naturally a year earlier; and when tested with smallpox variolation, he was immune. Case 4, Mary Barge, contracted cowpox naturally and then nursed several smallpox patients without contracting the disease. Case 5, Mrs. H., contracted cowpox when she was young and resisted both natural smallpox exposure and variolation with smallpox minor as an adult. Case 6, Sarah Wynne, contracted cowpox on her farm and, when she was naturally exposed to smallpox, didn't develop the disease. Case 7, William Rodway, caught cowpox naturally and was immune to smallpox afterward even though he was exposed to the disease several times.

Case 8, Elizabeth Wynne, contracted cowpox naturally years before and was immune when Jenner variolated her with smallpox minor. Case 9, William Smith, contracted cowpox three times and twice resisted variolation with smallpox minor. Case 10, Simon Nichols, contracted cowpox naturally and suffered no effects from variolation with smallpox minor. Case 11, William Stinchcombe, showed immunity to smallpox minor variolation after contracting cowpox naturally. Case 12 included several young females in a village near Jenner's home who were variolated with smallpox minor. He found that girls who had already contracted cowpox naturally were immune to variolation with smallpox minor while those who had not been naturally infected with cowpox contracted smallpox after variolation. Case 13, Thomas Pearce, caught horsepox naturally and was immune to variolation with smallpox minor. Case 14, James Cole also contracted horsepox and was immune to smallpox variolation. Case 15, Abraham Riddiford, caught horsepox naturally and was immune to variolation with smallpox minor.

In addition to the fifteen naturally occurring cases of cowpox infections that conferred immunity to smallpox, Jenner intentionally inoculated nine other children with serum taken from humans infected with cowpox and tested each of the inoculated children with smallpox minor variolation to determine if the intentional cowpox vaccine gave them immunity to smallpox.[126] On March 16, 1798, Jenner inoculated a five-year-old boy named John Baker with cowpox serum, and he developed symptoms of cowpox. John died from another contagious disease, most likely typhoid fever, which was rampant in England at the time before he could be variolated with smallpox minor. Jenner inoculated William Summers, aged five, with cowpox, variolated him with smallpox minor, and William developed no symptoms of smallpox.

Jenner took serum from a pustule on William's arm and inoculated a child named William Pead with cowpox. Pead developed cowpox, was variolated with smallpox minor, and developed no symptoms. William Pead provided serum to infect Hannah Excell, who developed cowpox pustules. Jenner used serum from Hannah to inoculate four more children. John Marklove, aged one-and-a-half years; Mary Pead, aged five; and Mary James, aged six, all developed symptoms of cowpox and were immune to smallpox minor variolation. The fourth child Jenner inoculated with serum from Hannah didn't develop any symptoms, so he must have been naturally immune from an earlier case of cowpox or smallpox. The final case of inoculation with cowpox serum was J. Barge, a seven-year-old who was infected with serum from Mary Pard. Jenner variolated J. Barge and an unvaccinated child with variola minor smallpox. J. Barge was immune to smallpox, but the other child developed symptoms of smallpox following variolation.

After collecting his cases of natural and intentional cowpox immunization and revising his paper, Jenner went to London with colored drawings of cowpox pustules as they occurred naturally on the milkmaids' hands or after inoculation with cowpox serum. He also brought dried cowpox serum from one of his children for use in London. Jenner intended to submit his paper to the Royal Society and use the dried serum to demonstrate his inoculation technique to London physicians.

Jenner's study of natural and artificial cowpox inoculations was accepted for publication by the Royal Society as an article titled *An Inquiry into the Causes and Effect of the Variolae Vaccinae, a Disease Discovered in Some of the Western Counties of England, Particularly Gloucestershire, and Known by the Name of Cow Pox.*[127] In early sections of his paper, Jenner described the inoculation method he had developed and the results discovered. In the last section, he explained the advantages of inoculation of children with cowpox as opposed to variolation with smallpox. Jenner argued that variolation with smallpox minor often caused scarring of the skin and death in 2 percent of children while no side effects or deaths occurred with cowpox inoculation. Moreover, Jenner said that cowpox inoculation could be performed without infecting other members of the family or the community, which was not true of variolation with smallpox. He pointed out that patients infected with variola minor smallpox could infect others.

He was unable to convince a single London physician to use his cowpox serum, so Jenner left the sample with Dr. Henry Cline, a friend and surgeon at St. Thomas Hospital. Cline decided to use the cowpox serum on one of his patients who had a hip problem, hoping the irritation caused by the cowpox would help the damaged hip. Cline inoculated his patient, who developed symptoms of cowpox, but the infection had no effect on the defective hip. Cline then decided to test Jenner's cowpox inoculation theory by variolating his patient with variola minor smallpox to see if he was immune. The patient resisted the smallpox infection, and Cline became an enthusiastic supporter of Jenner's cowpox vaccination.

His friend Cline and the king's physician, Sir Walter Farquhar, advised Jenner to open a medical practice of cowpox inoculations in London, saying he would make a fortune from the procedure. However, Jenner decided not to remain in London because he didn't believe he knew enough about how cowpox vaccination worked or the most effective methods of collecting, preparing, and storing cowpox serum. He had described his collection, storage, and inoculation procedures precisely in his article; but other physicians deviated from his methods, often producing poor results. A few of his medical colleagues followed his method carefully and produced confirming evidence that inoculation worked. A veterinary surgeon named Thomas Tanner infected cows with cowpox serum taken from humans who had contracted cowpox, showing that Jenner's theory that cowpox was a similar disease in cows and humans was correct. Another physician transferred cowpox to a child and then to a horse, verifying that the disease could travel between humans and other animals besides cows. However, there were also reported failures of Jenner's cowpox inoculation procedure.[128]

Problems with Cowpox Inoculation

Jenner's cowpox inoculation procedure sometimes failed to protect against smallpox while variolation with smallpox minor always succeeded in protecting a person from smallpox major if the child survived, and he didn't understand why. Jenner knew that smallpox minor variolation sometimes killed children while inoculation with cowpox was totally safe, but that didn't convince his fellow physicians. Another problem was that Jenner didn't know if the immunity induced by cowpox vaccination would last. Most puzzling to Jenner was the fact that not everyone who was inoculated with cowpox became immune to smallpox. His contemporaries suggested that the cause was different constitutions among his patients, but Jenner speculated that there were two types of cowpox, one that gave immunity to smallpox and another that didn't. After further study, he realized that cowpox serum had to be collected from an infected child at the proper time to be effective, and cowpox serum deteriorated over time if it was not stored correctly.[129] These two factors caused cowpox inoculation to now always work.

Proper Vaccination Procedure

Jenner found that when a cowpox vaccination caused eruptions on the patient's skin, the inoculation was always successful and the person was immune to smallpox; but when there were no skin eruptions, the inoculation might not have been successful, and he recommended it be repeated. Even today, if there is no reaction to a smallpox vaccine, it's repeated. He also discovered that the optimum time to take cowpox serum from a pustule was between the fifth and eighth days after it appeared. Before the fifth day, serum from the pustule contained too little cowpox virus to produce good immunity; and after the eighth day, the cowpox virus had begun to disappear from the serum and didn't reliably produce immunity to smallpox.

Jenner recommended a patient be reinoculated if there was concern that the procedure had not been effective and suggested that the best practice was to use fresh serum taken from an active pustule or cowpox serum stored no more than two or three days after it was collected. Older cowpox serum was often ineffective and caused failures.[130] He recommended placing serum on glass and allowing it to dry naturally but not to dry cowpox serum near the fire because heat killed the virus. After Jenner discovered the optimum time to collect cowpox serum from a pustule and how to store it properly, he was able to successfully immunize over one thousand patients with serum from a single child's cowpox infection with no failures. Jenner also discovered that in the rare cases when a child was inoculated with cowpox and later developed smallpox, the disease was always mild and the child never died.

Between January and May of 1799, Dr. William Woodville vaccinated six hundred children with cowpox serum and showed by smallpox variolation that all were immune to smallpox. Woodville published his findings in a pamphlet entitled *Report of a Series of Inoculations for the Variolae Vaccinae ... with Remarks and Observations of This Disease, Considered as a Substitute for the Small-Pox* in late May of 1799.[131] Woodville concluded that cowpox inoculation protected against smallpox, and he noted that cowpox pustules were different from smallpox pustules. In spite of the positive results reported for cowpox inoculations, opposition to the cowpox vaccine developed among physicians who were already using variolation to protect against smallpox because they had a financial interest in continuing the practice.

Opposition to Cowpox Inoculation

Criticism of Jenner's work by physicians at the Smallpox and Inoculation Hospital appeared soon after he published the *Inquiry.* The head of the hospital reported that among his patients, cowpox inoculation didn't protect against smallpox. After a careful review of the data from the Smallpox and Inoculation Hospital, modern physicians have concluded that the negative results from early cowpox inoculations at the hospital happened because patients vaccinated with cowpox were exposed to smallpox at the same time and probably contracted smallpox before the cowpox inoculations became effective.[132]

Ironically, George Pearson, head of the Smallpox and Inoculation Hospital, also claimed priority in discovering cowpox vaccination, which Jenner disputed.[133] Jenner accused Paterson of not inoculating his patients properly, pointing out that by administering cowpox vaccine in one arm and five days later, variolating the same patient in the other arm with smallpox didn't allow cowpox immunity to develop among these children before they developed smallpox, and that was why Peterson had produced confusing results. Jenner also noted that smallpox infections were prevalent in Peterson's hospital when he was vaccinating children with cowpox, so his results were doubly contaminated and necessarily inconclusive. After Jenner's criticisms of Paterson's procedures, the Duke of York withdrew his financial support from the Smallpox and Inoculation Hospital, and it closed.

The English royal family supported Jenner's work and the king invited him to dedicate a new edition of *Inquiry* to his royal person. He was received by the Prince of Wales and presented to Queen Charlotte. The queen's eighth son had died of smallpox variolation, so the prospect of a safe vaccine against smallpox held special meaning for her. Jenner successfully inoculated one of the queen's "protégés" named William, signaling solid social and political recognition of cowpox vaccination by the royal family. Having gained royal favor, Jenner moved to London for part of each year to practice cowpox inoculation and encourage other physicians to use the cowpox vaccine against smallpox. He reported that cowpox serum was always effective in inoculating patients against smallpox if it was collected at the proper time and stored correctly. Jenner offered free cowpox inoculations to poor families around Cheltenham, but one parish refused. Later, the villagers asked him for vaccinations because someone had contracted smallpox in the area.

In 1803, after the Napoleonic Wars began, the risk of smallpox epidemics within the English Army increased, so the Duke of York directed military medical governors to introduce cowpox vaccination in all their garrisons as soon as possible. The Royal Navy approved cowpox vaccination for sailors in 1800, and thousands of vaccinations were carried out in England and Scotland soon after.[134] However, the number of inoculations was small compared with the total population of the United Kingdom, so Jenner had a lot of work to do convincing Englishmen to get vaccinated. Jenner's reputation was growing throughout Europe, and he was beginning to collect awards and be recognized by other nations. Support for cowpox vaccination spread to Spain, Germany, Austro-Hungary, Holland, Denmark, and Sweden after 1800. On February 20, 1801, Jenner was given a gold medal by the medical officers of the Royal Navy for his discovery of cowpox inoculation. Jenner decided to file a petition with Parliament for compensation.

Conflict in Parliament

When Jenner presented his formal petition to Parliament for compensation, his old enemy George Pearson introduced evidence that contradicted some of Jenner's claims. Jenner said his contribution was showing that cowpox serum taken from one child could be used to inoculate another and perfecting the method of transferring cowpox serum from one child to another with no loss of effectiveness. Jenner told Parliament he had voluntarily disclosed his methods to the world, benefiting servicemen and the general public and stopping the spread of smallpox in England. In 1802, most members of the London medical community supported Jenner's claim that he had first discovered the efficacy of cowpox as a vaccine against smallpox, and Parliament voted to award Jenner ten thousand pounds for discovering the cowpox vaccine.[135] Soon after, his supporters passed a resolution establishing the Royal Jennerian Society to advance the use of cowpox inoculation throughout England.

The Royal Jennerian Society

The society received a five-hundred-pound donation from the Corporation of London, and its board of directors announced that the Bank of England and the East India Company would be recipients of all future donations.[136] The society established an inoculation center in London, and until a permanent inoculator could be found, members of the board worked in the clinic inoculating patients. They established a committee to hire a resident inoculator who would be responsible for vaccinating patients, collecting and storing cowpox serum, and sending samples of cowpox serum to other clinics. The inoculations were free to any resident of London. Dr. John Walker was selected as the first resident inoculator; and under his direction, the society vaccinated eleven hundred persons, supplied cowpox serum to over four hundred fifty inoculation clinics in London, and offered free cowpox serum to private practitioners throughout London. Other countries also began inoculation programs. For example, Paris vaccinated over sixty thousand children in 1803.

King Carlos of Spain ordered Dr. Francis X. Balmis to sail to India with twenty healthy children and one child who had active cowpox. The ship was ordered to stop at various ports, vaccinating children at each city where it anchored using live cowpox serum from an infected child. The medical party crossed Mexico by land and sailed to the Philippines with twenty-six healthy unvaccinated children and one child with cowpox on board. Over two hundred thirty thousand cowpox vaccinations were performed during the long voyage. However, English physicians who had been variolating patients continued to oppose cowpox inoculation for their own financial gain.

Opposition to Cowpox Inoculation

In 1805, an active campaign against cowpox vaccination developed in England.[137] Those opposing cowpox vaccination claimed it didn't always protect against smallpox, that variolation always protected against smallpox, and variolation didn't cause death (which was patently false because 2 percent of variolation patients died). The false claims against cowpox slowed the rate of cowpox inoculation in England, and fewer people were being vaccinated with cowpox each year while the number variolated with smallpox minor increased. Since variolated individuals were contagious, smallpox killed over six thousand persons in London in 1805. Opponents of cowpox vaccination even claimed it caused tuberculosis! Jenner responded that during his many years of vaccinating patients with cowpox serum, none had developed tuberculosis, and when cowpox vaccination was done properly, the patient was always protected against smallpox. His critics had financial reasons to criticize Jenner since they depended on smallpox variolation for their livelihood and continued to spread lies about the procedure.

While opponents of cowpox vaccination resorted to outright lies against the efficacy and side effects of the vaccine, other critics of Jenner argued that deaths from smallpox were a good thing because the country was going to run out of food if population growth was not curtailed. Jenner returned to London to defend cowpox inoculation against these scurrilous attacks. Also, he needed money because he had been spending over eight hundred pounds annually studying, promoting, and supplying free cowpox vaccinations. He planned to defend cowpox vaccinations and ask for another grant from Parliament while in London. Additionally, there was trouble at the Royal Jennerian Society because the board of directors was fighting among themselves.[138] Walker resigned soon after Jenner arrived in London, and later that year, the Jennerian Society closed.

The Royal College of Physicians issued a report on April 10, 1807, supporting the practice of cowpox vaccination to prevent smallpox, and Jenner received news that subscriptions in India had produced several hundred pounds for him. The funds were welcome because he needed money to promote the cowpox vaccine and continue his free clinics. On July 29, 1807, Parliament awarded Jenner an additional prize of twenty thousand pounds for his discovery and development of cowpox inoculation.[139] He returned to Cheltenham with his fortunes restored and the support of most Englishmen for his cowpox inoculation procedure. Jenner was fifty-eight years old and had reached the pinnacle of medical, financial, and social success when he was confronted with an apparent failure of the cowpox vaccine that threatened his life's work.

Vaccine Failure?

In late 1807, Jenner was asked to investigate an alleged failure of cowpox vaccination in Ringwood, a small village near his home. It was reported that a number of people had been vaccinated with cowpox, and several had contracted smallpox soon after. The number who died was uncertain but may have been as many as seventeen. A committee under Jenner's direction collected evidence about what had happened in the village. They found that on September 11, 1807, smallpox broke out in the village of Ringwood; and on October 16, seventy people were variolated with smallpox minor by two doctors in the area. The variolated individuals were told to stay away from other residents but were not placed in isolation. Village leaders allowed each resident to decide whether to undergo variolation with smallpox or receive a cowpox vaccination. In the rush to complete the two procedures, no one kept accurate records of who was inoculated with cowpox and who was variolated with smallpox minor, so the situation was totally confusing.

Jenner's committee published a report concluding that the smallpox infections among individuals who received cowpox inoculations most likely occurred because they had been exposed to smallpox prior to their cowpox vaccinations by the patients who had received smallpox variolations. The committee also noted that the dry serum used for cowpox inoculations had been placed in boiling water, which almost certainly rendered it ineffective before it was used. Finally, among the two cases who died after receiving the cowpox vaccine, one had a stroke and the other died from self-starvation. After the committee published its report, the antivaccine group was disgraced, and most physicians admitted that without proper quarantine, smallpox variolation spreads the disease while cowpox vaccination does not. Parliament began considering a bill to require the quarantine of individuals who had undergone smallpox variolation to protect neighbors from exposure to smallpox. Cowpox inoculation was now accepted as safe and effective by most Englishmen.

On June 9, 1808, the House of Commons passed a bill creating an institution in London to provide cowpox inoculations, supervised by the Royal College of Physicians and the Royal College of Surgeons. The institution was called the National Vaccine Establishment. Even as Parliament was supporting cowpox vaccination, critics claimed the immunity didn't last, so the inoculated person would get smallpox in the future. Jenner reported that the length of immunity varied with individuals, and some vaccinated persons did later catch smallpox. However, he pointed out that smallpox infections after inoculation with cowpox were always mild and not fatal while 2 percent of people variolated with smallpox minor died and 30 percent of uninoculated children infected with smallpox major died as a result of the infection.

In 1810, Jenner began experiencing roaring in his ears, heaviness in his muscles, and uncontrollable drowsiness, probably symptoms of depression following the death of his son Edward. Jenner was also torn between professional fame and family duties. His wife was ill, but his professional work kept him from home. He felt obligated to pay attention to his professional legacy because critics were still attacking cowpox vaccination, even in the face of overwhelming evidence that the procedure was safe and gave immunity against smallpox. However, he felt guilty about neglecting his family.

In support of cowpox vaccination, Robert Watt, a Glasgow physician, published statistics showing that deaths from smallpox among children younger than ten had fallen from almost 20 percent in 1783 to 4 percent by 1813 after the cowpox vaccine was introduced and became widely available. However, deaths from smallpox fluctuated from year to year, and Jenner was not certain why. He soon realized that the cyclic variations occurred because parents neglected to vaccinate their children when the threat of smallpox was low but vaccinated them when the threat of smallpox reappeared, causing cycles in the rate of smallpox deaths. Oxford University recognized Jenner for his work on vaccination in 1813.[140]

Dr. Jenner

The University of Oxford voted to award Jenner an honorary doctor of medicine degree; and on December 15, 1813, he received his diploma from Sir Christopher, regius professor of medicine at Oxford. Jenner was also presented to the vice-chancellor and several professors at Oxford. Now that he had a medical degree from Oxford, Jenner was eligible to become a fellow of the Royal College of Physicians. However, the college governors decided they would not admit Jenner without an examination, which would require him to relearn Latin and Greek. He was insulted and withdrew his application.

Jenner worked under several handicaps developing an effective cowpox vaccination. First, there was little formal regulation of physicians in London at the time, and many administered his vaccine improperly because they were not properly trained. Second, there was no standard way of differentiating one disease from another, except by observing symptoms. Third, there was no pharmaceutical industry capable of manufacturing a safe and effective vaccine in the early nineteenth century.[141] To inoculate his patients, Jenner had to transfer serum from one infected child to another because he could not manufacture and store a vaccine with available facilities. Fourth, there was no standard model for designing clinical trials, such as the double-blind randomized clinical trials used today, so physicians couldn't agree on what was a good test of the vaccine. Finally, medical journals were not peer-reviewed in the early nineteenth century, so anyone could criticize Jenner's work in print, whether the criticisms were valid or not. Given all these handicaps, it's remarkable Jenner was able to convince most of the world's medical community that cowpox inoculation was a safe and effective vaccine against smallpox. Humanity owes Edward Jenner a tremendous vote of thanks for saving literally hundreds of millions of people from smallpox by developing the cowpox vaccine.

Last Years

Jenner suffered a serious loss when his wife Catherine died on September 13, 1815. During the summer of 1820, he was walking in his garden when Jenner suddenly felt faint, fell, and was not discovered until hours later. He was put to bed, slept through the night, and felt fine the next morning. Apparently, he had suffered a mild stroke because he complained of lameness and inability to tolerate riding in a carriage because of motion sickness. He also complained that certain sounds, such as the striking of a bell, caused him to feel shocked. Concerned about his health, Jenner had a Berkeley attorney draft his will to protect members of his family who needed supervision and support.[142] Jenner gave his estate to his son Robert in trust for the support of his children or if Robert didn't marry, for the support of his daughter Catherine's children. Edward Jenner suffered a stroke on January 25, 1823, and died around two o'clock the following morning, January 26, 1823.

Chapter 7

---- ✝ ----

ANESTHETICS: WILLIAM MORTON

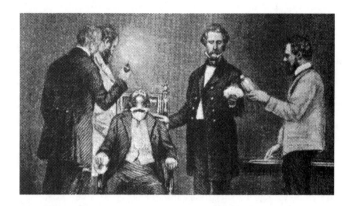

W illiam Morton attended a lecture on ether in a chemistry class at Harvard Medical School and wondered if the gas would allow surgeons and dentists to perform painless operations. He began studying the anesthetic effect of ether by administering it to animals. Next, Morton inhaled ether himself, felt lethargic, fell unconscious, and when he awakened, was certain he could have had a tooth extracted without experiencing any pain. He administered ether to some of his patients, confirmed it was safe, and arranged a demonstration of the anesthetic before Boston surgeons. Morton administered ether to a patient who experienced no pain during a surgical operation on his jaw. Attending doctors were impressed with Morton's anesthetic, and he was granted a patent by the US government for the discovery. Both Morton's former dental partner, Horace Wells, and his former Harvard chemistry professor, Charles Jackson, claimed they had discovered the anesthetic effects of ether before him. However, Harvard Medical School physicians supported Morton's claim of priority, and a congressional committee concluded that Morton had a good claim to the invention. He served as an army surgeon during the American Civil War, using ether to operate painlessly on hundreds of wounded Union soldiers.

William Morton was born on August 9, 1819, in Carlton, Minnesota. As a boy, he helped his father tap and drain maple trees, boil the sap into syrup, shear sheep, mow hay, and pick apples. He hunted and fished, skated on frozen ponds, and rode horses on the family farm. When he was eight, Morton entered Northfield and Leicester schools for a few years before his father went bankrupt and moved to Boston to work as a clerk, printer, and salesman. He entered Baltimore College of Dental Surgery, graduated in 1842, and formed a dental partnership with Horace Wells in Boston.[143] While they were partners, Wells began experimenting with nitrous oxide as an anesthetic. Surgeons and dentists had been searching for a safe and effective anesthetic for centuries, but none had been found.

Search for an Anesthetic

Historians believe the first substance used to relieve pain was opium, extracted from poppies by the Mesopotamians around 5,000 BC.[144] The anesthetic effect of cannabis was described by Homer and known to ancient Chinese physicians. European mandrake was used to suppress pain during amputations in the sixteenth century, and during the eighteenth century, Franz Mesmer developed the process of hypnosis, or animal magnetism as he called the technique, which he claimed produced insensitivity to pain. A few surgeons and dentists employed hypnosis in their practices, but most believed the technique was impractical because it required too much time to induce the desired mental state, and only some persons were susceptible.

In 1799, Sir Humphrey Davies experimented with nitrous oxide and published a report stating that the gas relieved the pain of a toothache or headache when inhaled. Davies also suggested that nitrous oxide might be used during surgery to relieve pain, but never pursued the matter.[145] Horace Wells may have read Davies's article on nitrous oxide before beginning his studies of nitrous oxide as an anesthetic. The inhalation of ether to suppress pain in the chest was suggested by Richard Pearson in 1795; and Dr. John Warren, an American physician, recommended the inhalation of ether to relieve inflammation of the lungs. James Y. Simpson discovered the anesthetic effects of chloroform in 1847, a year after Morton demonstrated that ether can be used to perform painless dentistry and surgery.[146] Many physicians concluded that chloroform, which caused blistering of the skin and sickness in many patients, had too many side effects to be a useful anesthetic and rejected it as a safe and effective anesthetic during surgery and dentistry. Horace Wells was interested in finding a way to perform painless dentistry when he began experimenting with nitrous oxide.

Nitrous Oxide

Wells recognized its anesthetic effects during a public demonstration in which Gardner Colton administered nitrous oxide to Samuel Cooley.[147] Wells noticed that while Cooley was under the influence of nitrous oxide, he struck his leg hard against a bench but showed no sign he experienced any pain. Wells thought nitrous oxide might be the anesthetic he was searching for and asked John Riggs to extract one of his teeth while under the influence of the gas. After the extraction, Wells reported he felt no pain from the dental procedure and believed nitrous oxide was a safe and effective anesthetic for use in surgery and dentistry. However, his discovery was rejected by the Boston medical and dental communities after a public demonstration of the pain-killing effect of nitrous oxide scheduled at Massachusetts General Hospital in January of 1845 failed.

While under the influence of nitrous oxide, Wells's patient groaned during the surgical operation, causing observers to conclude he felt pain and that nitrous oxide was not an effective anesthetic. Morton and Wells dissolved their partnership soon after the failure of his demonstration of nitrous oxide. Soon after he split with Wells, Morton fell in love with Elizabeth Whitman, but her family opposed the marriage because he was a dentist. Morton agreed to attend medical school if her family approved the marriage, and he entered Harvard Medical School in 1844 to become a doctor.[148]

Medical School

Morton attended anatomy classes, dissected human cadavers, studied chemistry, and listened to lectures on midwifery during his first year at Harvard. He also took classes on the practice of medicine, learned to treat patients, recognize the symptoms of various diseases, and perform surgery. In addition to taking classes, Harvard medical students were required to accompany practicing physicians and surgeons as they treated patients and performed surgeries at Massachusetts General Hospital, the leading hospital in Boston at that time and a pioneer in medicine and surgery. However, before the use of ether was introduced to render a patient unconscious during surgery, cuts by a scalpel triggered such agonized screams from patients that two strong assistants were required to hold a patient down until the surgery was finished and the patient could be taken, weak and bloodied, to a recovery room. Morton was shocked by the ordeal patients endured during surgery and became interested in finding a safe and effective anesthetic well before he attended a fateful class in chemistry given by Professor Charles T. Jackson.

Professor Jackson

During his time at Harvard Medical School, Morton attended a chemistry lecture given by Professor Charles Jackson, who discussed the anesthetic properties of ether in one of his lectures and speculated that it might be an effective anesthetic for use during surgery.[149] Jackson never took any steps to demonstrate ether was a safe and effective anesthetic for use on human patients during surgery or dentistry, so he lost priority for the discovery of ether as an anesthetic to Morton who demonstrated that surgery could be painless under the influence of ether. Morton left medical school without graduating and returned to his dental practice in 1844 because he needed money. In his dental practice, Morton specialized in fitting artificial teeth and developed a process that avoided the problems of bad breath and sour taste caused by regular artificial teeth used at the time. The procedure for fitting an artificial tooth at that time was to fasten a gold plate over the root of a decayed tooth and solder an artificial tooth to the gold plate with a soft solder so the heat from soldering would not melt the gold plate. The problem with this procedure was that the gold plate and soft solder generated a small electric current when immersed in saliva, turning the solder black, creating an unsightly dark line between the tooth and gum, causing a bad odor and introducing a sour taste in the patient's mouth.

Morton claimed he could avoid the black line, bad odor, and sour taste by extracting the patient's tooth, installing a gold plate in the patient's mouth affixed to the teeth next to the artificial tooth, and using a gold solder that didn't create an electrical current to affix the new false tooth to the gold plate.[150] However, extracting a tooth was painful at that time, so many patients declined Dr. Morton's procedure. Morton realized he needed some way to avoid the pain caused by tooth extraction if he wanted to increase the income from his dental practice and began searching for a safe and effective anesthetic. He tried brandy, champagne, laudanum, opium, and hypnosis as anesthetics with little success. The alcohol didn't eliminate pain, laudanum and opium often made patients sick, and many of his dental patients couldn't be hypnotized. In spite of his failures, Morton continued to search for a substance that would anesthetize his patients and allow him to perform dental procedures without causing pain. Another problem Morton faced was that he needed a ready supply of artificial teeth, and none was available in Boston. To fulfill his own need for artificial teeth and increase his income, Morton established a factory to manufacture artificial teeth for his own practice and distributed them to dentists in America and Europe.

Manufacturing Artificial Teeth

The first step in manufacturing artificial teeth was to grind quartz and spar stone into a fine powder, using a steam engine and grinding wheel.[151]

Next, workers mixed metallic oxides and liquids with the powdered stone to create a paste that was used to fill small die and form the artificial teeth. Female workers filled tooth-shaped dies with paste, allowed it to dry, and then opened the dies to produce natural-shaped artificial teeth made of ground quartz, spar stone, and metallic oxides. These artificial teeth were polished to make them smooth and placed in a furnace to harden before a platina pin was inserted in the bottom of each tooth (platina is an alloy of platinum, palladium, osmium, and iridium) so it could be attached to the root of a person's tooth. Enamel was applied to the artificial teeth with a camel hair brush to make them appear natural, and the finished teeth were placed in a coal-fired furnace to bake a second time and harden the enamel to produce natural-looking artificial teeth. While Morton was setting up his artificial tooth factory and practicing dentistry, he recalled what Professor Jackson had said about ether being an anesthetic that might allow painless surgery and decided to meet with him and discuss the topic in detail.

Experimenting with Ether

When Morton met with Professor Jackson to discuss the anesthetic effects of ether, he encouraged Morton to experiment and determine whether ether would work clinically and allow surgeons or dentists to perform painless operations or extractions. Morton began by studying what was already known about the anesthetic effects of ether in the summer of 1846.[152] He read several published articles about the effects of ether and discovered it was capable of intoxicating a patient when inhaled and was used to treat pulmonary pain. He consulted with chemists about the properties of ether and discussed the best way of administering ether to patients while planning how to test whether ether might be an effective anesthetic and allow dentists and surgeons to perform painless operations and tooth extractions.

Morton began studying ether by administering the gas to animals, hoping to show it was safe and effective. He also applied liquid ether to some of his patients' teeth to see if it would numb the pain of a toothache.

Applying liquid ether to a tooth turned out to be time-consuming and tedious, so Morton decided to see if inhaling ether would produce effective pain relief and anesthesia. He experimented on animals, himself, and a few patients to prove inhaling ether was safe and blocked pain. He needed to be careful because the articles discussing ether warned of serious side effects if too much of the gas was inhaled by a patient. One book suggested that some patients, who were particularly susceptible to ether, could experience stupefaction for periods of up to thirty hours after inhaling the gas. Other articles reported that patients who showed a lowered pulse rate while inhaling ether might even die after inhaling it. Morton concluded that ether was safe if administered in moderate quantities, but at high doses, it could be life-threatening, so he needed to be careful about how much he gave each patient. He set out to determine the amount of ether that constituted a safe dose in human patients and see if that dose was adequate to produce an anesthetic effect.[153]

Morton also tested to see if combining a narcotic, such as opium, with ether might make the gas more effective as an anesthetic; he breathed ether and morphine through a warm towel to test the effect. The combination of ether and morphine produced a general feeling of numbness but caused Morton to suffer a severe headache, so he abandoned the idea. In the spring of 1846, Thomas R. Spear joined Morton's dental practice as a student and told Morton he had often inhaled pure ether and never experienced any adverse side effects from the gas. This comment by Spear made Morton wonder if perhaps the ether he was using was impure and the impurities were causing the negative side effects he was experiencing. Morton decided to have a chemist analyze a sample of the ether he had been using and let him know if it contained impurities. The chemist Morton consulted said he knew of people who inhaled ether, became exhilarated, hurt themselves, but experienced no pain while under its influence. He also warned Morton that too large a dose of ether could kill a patient. The chemist analyzed Morton's ether and found it contained small amounts of impurities and substantial quantities of alcohol. Morton decided he needed to find a source of pure ether to use in his work so he could avoid negative side effects.[154]

Pure Ether

Morton was able to purchase a bottle of pure sulfuric ether from a chemist to use in his experiments on animals to determine if it produced any side effects, to discover the proper dose for inducing unconsciousness and how to avoid killing his patient. He poured pure ether on a cotton pad, placed it at the bottom of a pan, and held a dog's head directly above the pan while the animal breathed the ether fumes. In a few minutes, the animal fell unconscious and could not be aroused by pinching. When Morton moved the ether away from the dog's nose, it recovered consciousness in about three minutes and showed no ill effects from inhaling the pure ether. Morton wondered if the same effect could be produced in a human being and decided to try inhaling pure ether himself and see what happened.

As an initial test to determine whether pure ether was safe for humans to breathe, Morton soaked a small amount of ether in a handkerchief and inhaled the fumes himself. He became unconscious in a few minutes, and when Morton awakened, he felt certain he would not have felt any pain while unconscious.[155] He next administered pure ether to some of his patients to make certain inhaling it was safe, induced unconsciousness, and caused no serious side effects. Convinced he had made an important discovery, Morton became concerned that others might try to steal his idea and claim it as their own, so he became secretive about what he was doing. He decided to have his students purchase ether from a manufacturer rather than buying it himself from a pharmacy to hide his identity and purpose from potential competitors.

However, when Morton used the ether bought by his students, his patients became excited and aroused rather than calm and unconscious. He immediately decided the ether his students had bought was impure, so he had it analyzed by a chemist, who discovered it contained a large amount of alcohol. Morton decided in the future he would have ether analyzed for purity before using it on patients because only pure ether seemed to be a safe and effective anesthetic that produced no negative side effects. Now that he knew impurities were causing the negative side effects his patients had experienced when inhaling ether, Morton felt certain he had discovered a safe and effective anesthetic and set out to design an apparatus to administer the gas to his patients.

Administering Ether

Morton discussed how to design and construct an apparatus to administer ether to patients with Joseph M. Wightman, a scientific instrument maker. Based on these discussions, Morton bought a glass globe with two openings, placed a sponge soaked in ether in the globe, and had his patients inhale the ether fumes through one of the openings. By inhaling the mixture of ether and air through one opening of the glass globe, his patients were able to absorb sufficient quantities of pure ether to render them unconscious without receiving too large a dose that might put them at risk of dying. Morton purchased a quantity of pure ether and experimented on himself by inhaling ether and air from the glass globe. For some reason, the technique didn't work for Morton, so he poured pure ether on his handkerchief and inhaled that while looking at his watch. Morton lost consciousness breathing ether through his handkerchief and, when he recovered, felt numbness in his limbs.[156] He pinched himself in several places and found he had no sensation of pain. Checking his watch, Morton discovered he had been unconscious for about eight minutes, which he believed was adequate time to perform a tooth extraction or simple surgical operation. He felt ready to try his new anesthetic on some of his dental patients.

Painless Dentistry

On September 30, 1846, Morton extracted a tooth from Eben H. Frost after administering pure ether to render him unconscious, demonstrating for the first time that painless dentistry was possible. Mr. Frost signed an affidavit that he had experienced no pain from a tooth extraction while under the influence of ether. A. G. Tenney and G. Hayden witnessed the affidavit confirming Morton had performed the painless extraction of a tooth under the influence of ether. During the procedure, Mr. Frost became unconscious after breathing pure ether and air for a little over one minute, felt no pain during the tooth extraction, and suffered no side effects when he recovered consciousness. Morton experimented with other patients and found that some of them remained conscious after inhaling the ether but were insensitive to pain, and he could extract a tooth without causing any pain. He found that some patients required four or five minutes of inhaling ether before they became unconscious and a tooth could be extracted painlessly while other patients fell unconscious in one or two minutes. Morton's success in performing painless dentistry was reported in the *Boston Daily Journal* on October 1, 1846, and created a sensation in the dental and medical community. His use of ether as an anesthetic was reported in several New England papers, and the Boston medical community became interested in his procedure for use during surgical operations. Morton refused to disclose the specific substance he was using to render his patients unconscious but agreed to demonstrate the procedure to surgeons at Massachusetts General Hospital.

Public Demonstration of Ether

Dr. Henry Bigelow, a professor of surgery at Harvard Medical School, suggested he and Morton arrange a public demonstration of the anesthetic properties of the substance he was using at Massachusetts General Hospital. Morton agreed to schedule a public demonstration on October 16, 1846, in the operating theater at the hospital and offered to administer the undisclosed substance (pure ether) to a patient to induce unconsciousness before a hospital surgeon performed the operation.[157] On the day scheduled for the operation, Morton arrived at the operating theater, introduced himself to the patient, and assured the man he would feel no pain during surgery. Morton administered ether to the patient, who fell unconscious in approximately five minutes. The medical audience was silent and paid close attention during the demonstration. Morton turned to Dr. Warren, the surgeon scheduled to perform the operation, and announced that his patient was ready for the procedure to begin. Dr. Warren made an incision in the skin of his patient and proceeded to remove a large tumor from the jaw. The patient made no sound and didn't move during the operation. When the surgery was complete, Dr. Warren stitched the surgical wound closed, washed the patient's face, bandaged him, and waited for the man to regain consciousness. When he regained consciousness, the surgeon asked if he felt any pain, and the patient said, "No, I felt only a sensation like scraping with a blunt instrument." Dr. Warren turned to the audience and announced, "Gentlemen! This is no humbug."[158]

The Boston surgeons observing the first painless operation were impressed with Morton's demonstration of ether as an anesthetic. Dr. Warren, the surgeon who performed the initial painless operation, asked Morton if he would administer the anesthetic to another patient the next day. Morton agreed, and scheduling arrangements were made. The following day, Morton administered ether to a young woman, and she remained unconscious and quiet while a large tumor was removed from her arm without pain. After these two operations, the practice of administering ether to surgical patients was discontinued at Massachusetts General Hospital because the trustees said they needed to know what substance Morton was using to induce unconsciousness in the patients before they would allow any more painless surgical operations at their hospital. Morton wrote a letter to Dr. Warren saying he was willing to share that information with the surgeons, but only if they would keep it in strict confidence because he was applying for a patent and didn't want someone else to apply before him. Morton also offered to train others in the use of ether as an anesthetic for reasonable compensation.

Dr. Henry Bigelow asked Morton to accompany him to Massachusetts General Hospital the next day where they discussed the matter with the hospital trustees.[159] Morton was told by the trustees that he could not use his procedure at the hospital if he would not publicly disclose what substance he was using to induce unconsciousness because the hospital had a strict rule against using secret remedies. Morton agreed to their terms and went to the operating room with Dr. Bigelow to inform the surgeons gathered there that he was using pure sulfuric ether as an anesthetic and he hoped the surgeons would allow him to continue administering it to patients so they could operate without pain. The surgeons said they wanted to continue using ether because it was painless for their patients, and now that they knew what Morton was using, he could continue administering the anesthetic. Over the next few months, several painless surgical operations were performed at Massachusetts General Hospital, with Morton in charge of administering the ether. He published the results of these painless surgical operations in medical journals and shared his technical procedures with the medical and dental communities of Boston.

A few days after Morton's meeting with the trustees of Massachusetts General Hospital, Professor Jackson from Harvard Medical School appeared at the hospital with a small container of oxygen and told the surgeons that oxygen should always be available when administering ether because the anesthetic might kill patients if they inhaled too much, but pure oxygen could revive them before they died. The surgeons were skeptical of his claim because Jackson was a chemist rather than a surgeon and was neither familiar with surgical procedures nor the effects of ether on surgical patients. Moreover, Jackson had a history of disputing the priority of inventors, having claimed he had given Samuel F. B. Morse the idea for the telegraph in 1832. Leaders in the Boston medical community agreed that merely suggesting an idea, without carrying out the experiments necessary to demonstrate the invention actually worked, was not sufficient evidence to support a claim that Jackson or anyone else had discovered the anesthetic effects of ether before Morton. Jackson's comments did raise concerns about the safety of ether as a general anesthetic for patients, however.

Safety Concerns

Surgeons in the Massachusetts area began to wonder if ether was safe to use on their patients because they knew earlier studies of the gas had produced mixed results. However, after additional public demonstrations of ether as a safe and effective anesthetic at the Massachusetts General Hospital and testimonials from several prominent physicians and surgeons, most doctors came to believe pure ether was safe when used according to Morton's careful procedures. Surgeons in Europe also tested pure ether as an anesthetic and found it safe and effective. However, a group of dentists in Boston, led by J. F. Flagg, opposed the use of ether in dentistry, reporting that many young women who inhaled the gas suffered bleeding of the lungs, depression, and delirium afterward. Morton responded to these claims by arguing that the negative side effects of ether on these patients were caused by impure ether, and if they had used pure ether as he recommended, it was a safe and effective anesthetic.

Edward Warren, a nephew of Dr. Warren (the surgeon who had performed the first painless operation at Massachusetts General Hospital using ether as an anesthetic), traveled to Washington, DC, on Morton's behalf to introduce ether to US Army and Navy leaders. America was fighting a war with Mexico at the time, the services were suffering casualties, and Morton wanted to offer his discovery as a painless way to operate on wounded soldiers and sailors. The US Navy Bureau of Medicine and Surgery concluded that using ether in large hospitals may be justified, but it was too expensive to use on ships. The acting surgeon general of the United States wrote that because ether was highly volatile, it was not adapted to the difficult conditions of an army field hospital, and he could not recommend its use as an anesthetic on soldiers in the field. Morton was surprised and discouraged by these rejections, but decided to pursue his quest for a patent anyway. He contacted a patent attorney in Boston to discuss the idea of applying for a patent on ether as an anesthetic.

US Patent

Morton always claimed he filed for a patent on ether as an anesthetic so he could control the quality of the ether used in surgery and dentistry and train qualified doctors and dentists in proper procedures for its use. He reminded his critics that he had experienced several failures using impure ether during his early studies on animals and wanted to make certain only pure sulfuric ether was used as an anesthetic and was made available to qualified surgeons and dentists who could be counted on to use the anesthetic properly. Morton also said he would make his invention available without restrictions to qualified surgeons and dentists in good faith, citing his prior disclosure that he was using pure sulfuric ether as an anesthetic to the trustees and surgeons at Massachusetts General Hospital as proof of his good intentions. Morton engaged Richard H. Eddy, a patent attorney in Boston, to evaluate his claim for a patent on the use of pure sulfuric ether as an anesthetic. Eddy told Morton he doubted the idea was patentable but promised to review the evidence and give him a formal opinion soon. After three weeks, Eddy said he believed a patent could be obtained for the discovery, and Morton authorized him to file an application with the United States Patent and Trademark Office on his behalf.

On November 12, 1846, Morton's patent, number 4848, for the discovery of pure sulfuric ether as an anesthetic was approved by US secretary of state James Buchanan. The patent was issued to Morton as the discoverer, and Jackson as his adviser, for fourteen years. Morton began selling licenses for the use of ether as an anesthetic to physicians for $850. His patent attorney sailed to England to apply for a patent in that country after contracting with an English citizen to procure the patent and assign it to Morton for a fee. Morton's patent attorney also submitted applications covering the use of pure sulfuric ether as an anesthetic to the governments of Russia, Austria, France, Belgium, Sweden, Denmark, Saxony, Hanover, Holland, and Bavaria. Morton offered free licenses for the use of his patent to charitable institutions and sent samples of his inhaling apparatus and detailed instructions for its use to prominent physicians and dentists in the US so they could administer ether to their patients using his procedure. Morton offered to sell his apparatus to any qualified dentist or surgeon in the country and train him in its use.

Morton contracted with several medical apparatus manufacturers to produce and distribute his ether inhaling apparatus. He also conferred with Dr. Oliver W. Holmes Sr. about what to call the state a patient experienced under the influence of ether. They decided the word "anesthesia" was appropriate for the state of unconsciousness induced by ether. It didn't take long after the use of ether became widespread in America before others began claiming they had discovered the anesthetic properties of ether before Morton.

Prior Claims

After Morton published his studies showing pure sulfuric ether was an effective anesthetic and could be safely used to perform painless dentistry and surgery, disputes arose over who first discovered ether as an effective anesthetic. Dr. Horace Wells and Professor Charles Jackson each claimed they had discovered the anesthetic effect of ether prior to Morton. However, leaders in government, medicine, and dentistry quickly concluded there was little doubt William Morton had first publicly demonstrated the anesthetic effect of pure sulfuric ether by arranging with Drs. Bigelow and Warren to perform painless public surgeries at Massachusetts General Hospital. The only person who had performed painless surgery using ether as an anesthetic prior to Morton in 1846 was Crawford Long of Georgia, and he neither published nor disclosed his results until years after Morton publicly demonstrated the efficacy of ether so his priority didn't count.

Dr. H. J. Bigelow, professor of surgery at Harvard Medical School, who arranged the original demonstration of ether as an anesthetic at Massachusetts General Hospital, issued a public letter supporting Morton's claim of priority. Dr. Bigelow said in his public letter that Morton was the first person to prove ether was a safe and effective anesthetic that could be used in surgical operations to relieve pain. Bigelow also stated in his public letter that Professor Jackson's suggestion in class that ether might be an anesthetic was not sufficient to give him a prior claim because the professor had done nothing to prove ether was a safe and effective anesthetic for use with human patients. Bigelow argued that public proof of safety and efficacy were the hallmarks of an invention and essential to claim priority.[160] Simply suggesting that an idea might work was insufficient, in Dr. Bigelow's opinion, to support Jackson's claim to be the first discoverer of ether.

After Bigelow made his letter public, Jackson wrote to Morton requesting he be paid $500 for medical instruction concerning the use of ether as an anesthetic, hoping to profit from his association with Morton in medical school. Morton agreed to assign Professor Jackson 10 percent of any net profits from his patent if it amounted to as much as $500. Jackson based his claim for compensation on the fact that he supervised Morton as a medical student at Harvard in 1844 and lectured on the effectiveness of ether as an anesthetic in his chemistry class. Mr. Eddy, as part of his due diligence concerning the US patent, had asked Professor Jackson if he had done any experiments with ether as an anesthetic, and Professor Jackson said he had not. Mr. Eddy advised Morton that having Professor Jackson's name associated with the patent as an adviser would improve its chance of being issued, and Morton agreed to list Jackson as his adviser on the patent to increase its chance of being granted. Morton also decided to ask Congress to compensate him for the discovery of ether as an anesthetic in return for giving the government free use of his patent.

Congressional Compensation

Morton filed a request for compensation with Congress for his discovery of ether as an anesthetic, and several House members supported the application, saying the US government had paid inventors for the use of their ideas in the past.[161] On December 28, 1846, Edward Warren presented a formal application to Congress on behalf of Morton for compensation of his discovery that ether is a safe and effective anesthetic. The application was referred to a select congressional committee for review and recommendation. Congressman Dixon, the representative from the Connecticut district where Dr. Wells lived, protested the application before the select committee and asked members to receive evidence from Dr. Wells about his prior discovery of ether. Professor Jackson wrote to Congress stating that the claim by Dr. Wells was false, and the committee dropped Wells's claim.

Trustees of Massachusetts General Hospital issued a formal report stating that Dr. Morton had first discovered that pure ether could be safely and effectively used to induce anesthesia in surgical patients and that Professor Jackson had only made suggestions about ether as an anesthetic without any proof it was safe or effective in inducing an anesthetic state in patients. After Jackson learned there would be no profit from Morton's patent, he rejected the agreement with Morton for a percentage of the net profits from the invention, renewed his claim to be the original discoverer of ether as an anesthetic, and said he had been swindled by Morton. Jackson also said he would offer the discovery of ether as an anesthetic free to all medical men so he could gain favor with the medical community and disparage Morton. Jackson didn't disclose to the medical community that he had learned a few days earlier his agreement with Morton was worthless and that he had voided the agreement to receive 10 percent of the royalties from Morton's patent the day before, misleading doctors and dentists about his motives.

Despite strong support from the trustees of Massachusetts General Hospital and Dr. Bigelow, Congress declined to award Morton any compensation for his discovery. The congressional standing committee issued a report in 1849, stating that after a careful review of Morton's claims concerning the discovery of ether, he was entitled to the "merit of his discovery." The committee report also concluded that Professor Jackson may have had the idea that ether might be an anesthetic, but did not carry out the necessary studies to show it was safe and effective, so he had no prior claim to the patent. The congressional report also stated that the committee was greatly impressed by the report from the trustees of Massachusetts General Hospital that Morton was the sole discoverer of ether as an anesthetic, but declined to award Morton any compensation for the use of his patent by the US government.[162]

In 1851, Morton traveled to Washington personally to request compensation for his discovery of ether a second time and conferred with Secretary of State Daniel Webster about how to proceed.[163] Webster advised Morton to resubmit his claim to a select committee of Congress for consideration and see what happened. The second select committee concluded that before September 30, 1846, it was not known that pure sulfuric ether would induce anesthesia in a patient, sufficient to produce insensibility to pain. After Morton's demonstration, the committee stated there was no doubt ether was safe and effective, and Dr. Morton was the first person to show its anesthetic effect. The select committee recommended that Congress award Dr. Morton $100,000 as a reward for his discovery of ether as an anesthetic. The committee also recommended amending a defense appropriation bill to authorize $100,000 for the person whom a committee of three distinguished scientists appointed by the president determines is the discoverer of ether. The amendment failed, so Morton never received a penny from Congress for discovering the anesthetic effect of ether. He was also accused of criminal activities by jealous doctors and dentists.

Some of his enemies alleged that between 1835 and 1841, when Morton lived in Rochester, Cincinnati, St Louis, New Orleans, and Baltimore, he embezzled money, stole goods, and forged documents before fleeing to avoid arrest.[164] These allegations were never proved, and it seems likely rivals were trying to slander his reputation and claim prior discovery of the anesthetic effects of ether for themselves years later.

Last Years

The operating theater at Massachusetts General Hospital, where the first public demonstration of the anesthetic effects of ether occurred, has been turned into a monument to Dr. William Morton and is called the Ether Dome. In 1852, Morton was awarded an honorary degree of doctor of medicine by Washington University, and he volunteered to enter the US Army as a surgeon during the American Civil War and successfully administered ether to thousands of wounded Union soldiers while he performed the surgery.[165] He died on July 15, 1868, of a stroke in New York City.

Chapter 8

ANTISEPTIC SURGERY: JOSEPH LISTER

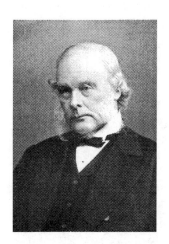

Wile in medical school, Lister became interested in the cause of hospital infections and how to avoid them, so he began collecting pus from infected wounds to examine under his microscope. He saw small creatures in the pus and wondered if hospital infections might be caused by germs that contaminated patients' wounds, causing illness and death. He eventually decided to search for an antiseptic that would destroy the small organisms he was seeing in his microscope before they killed his patients. Lister found that carbolic acid killed germs but didn't damage surrounding tissue and recommended surgeons bathe wounds in carbolic acid to kill germs and avoid postoperative infections. He found that mortality rates dropped from 45 percent to 15 percent among his hospital patients after Lister began using carbolic acid as an antiseptic in the hospital. Because of his work, antiseptics saved countless lives during surgery and childbirth decades before antibiotics became available to fight infections.

Joseph Lister was born on April 5, 1827, in London, England. He learned how to use the microscope from his father, who invented a lens in 1830 to correct chromatic aberration (a distortion of magnified images caused by light of different colors being bent in different amounts when passing through a glass lens). Lister's Quaker family was surprised when he announced he wanted to be a surgeon since no one in the family had ever been a doctor. He entered University College London at the age of seventeen because it had no religious requirements, which allowed him to enroll without being a member of the Church of England.[166] He completed an arts degree before entering medical school, which was unusual at the time—most students went directly to medical school.

While in medical school, Lister began studying tissue from infected patients under his microscope and saw small organisms in the samples he collected. Lister wondered if these small creatures were causing infections and speculated that if he could find a way to kill these small organisms, he might be able to prevent surgical infections and save lives. First, he needed to finish medical school.[167] University College London Medical School taught anatomy by dissection, but the cadavers decomposed quickly and the dissecting room smelled terrible. Dissecting dead bodies was not only unpleasant but also carried a serious risk of death for medical students. Professors warned their students that even a small cut during dissection could be fatal if it became infected. Between dead cadavers and diseased patients, the lifespan of a medical student could be short. Forty-one medical students died from infections between 1843 and 1859 at St. Bartholomew's Hospital alone.

Lister developed smallpox while in medical school and survived, but he became depressed and considered withdrawing to study for the ministry. Lister's father advised him to stay with medicine and do God's work. To overcome his depression, Lister traveled to the Isle of Wright, visited Ireland, and spent a year touring England and the continent before returning to medical school. After finishing his medical training, Lister began a residency at University College Hospital in 1850.[168] A few months later, he was offered the position of assistant to John Eric Erichsen, the hospital's senior surgeon. London hospitals were called "death houses" by the public because they were overcrowded, dirty, and breeding grounds for disease. Infection was so likely following surgery that only the most urgent cases were sent to the operating room as a last resort. Physicians and surgeons believed there was little anyone could do about infections, but Lister didn't agree. He believed unsanitary conditions in hospital wards and operating rooms were causing many of these infections and wanted to find a way to prevent them.

Causes of Infection

Some physicians had suggested that infections were caused by chemicals floating in the air, but no one knew how diseases were transmitted from patient to patient or how to stop their spread. James Y. Simpson compared the mortality rate of patients who underwent surgery in the country with those who endured surgery in city hospitals and found that among amputations performed in the country, 30 percent died while among patients who underwent amputations in the Royal Infirmary of Edinburgh, 91 percent died.[169] The main causes of death for amputees in the country were shock and exhaustion while deaths among amputees in the city hospital were caused mostly by infections. After reading these results, Lister became more determined to find out what caused hospital infections and how to prevent them.

William Sharpey, a Scottish professor of physiology and expert at using a microscope to study disease, became Lister's mentor at University College Hospital. He encouraged Lister to continue searching for a way to stop hospital infections. In 1852, gangrene began spreading through the hospital, and Lister was assigned to treat these patients. He scraped brown pus from their limbs while they were anesthetized and treated the cleaned wounds with a compound of mercury pernitrate before bandaging them. Many of the wounds healed as a result of his treatment. Lister was encouraged and renewed his effort to understand what was causing infections and how to avoid them. He prepared slides of the pus collected from patients' wounds, studied the slides under his microscope, and made sketches of the creatures he observed in his slides.[170] Lister concluded that the small creatures he was observing were causing gangrene, thought they were probably parasites, but he didn't know how to kill them. He began systematically searching for a chemical that would kill the small creatures and avoid infections among his patients. However, his independent attitude offended many professors.

During his residency, Lister earned several awards, but his professors were upset because he didn't automatically accept their teachings as true if he had seen contradictory evidence through his microscope. Because of his independence, Lister was often placed at the bottom of the honors list even though he was the best student in the entire class. Lister considered becoming a practicing surgeon but decided he wanted to understand how to kill the small organisms he observed in pus from infected wounds before they killed his patients. After completing his residency, Lister became a clinical clerk to the senior physician at University College Hospital and began looking for a position where he could pursue research. His mentor, Professor Sharpey, recommended Lister work with his friend, James Syme, in Scotland.

Collaboration with Syme

Sharpey suggested that Lister might want to spend a year learning what physicians and surgeons on the continent were doing about infections, or he could work on hospital infections in Scotland with his friend James Syme, professor of surgery at the University of Edinburgh.[171] Sharpey said Syme would be an excellent mentor for Lister, and they could work together researching infections and antiseptics. Lister wanted to meet Syme before he made up his mind, so in September 1853, he traveled to Edinburgh with a letter of introduction from Sharpey. Lister learned that Syme managed three wards at the Royal Infirmary, and he could gain valuable experience treating infected surgical patients. He liked Syme, who invited Lister to be his assistant and asked him to compile his clinical lectures so they could be published in the *Monthly Journal of Medical Science*. Lister joined Syme and included some of his own research on the cellular structure of bone tumors in these publications. In January 1854, Lister was officially appointed house surgeon by Syme, a job he had been doing for some time. Since Lister was not licensed to practice surgery in Scotland, he could assist Syme in the operating room, but could not perform surgery on his own. He advanced rapidly at the hospital because England was at war in Crimea, and many young surgeons were dying of disease in the army hospitals.

Crimean War

In 1853, the Crimean War began, and many young English surgeons died of cholera while treating soldiers in military hospitals.[172] As a result, Lister, who could not participate in the war because of his Quaker religion, advanced quickly as surgical positions opened due to the premature deaths of senior surgeons. Lister decided he wanted to lecture on surgery and become Syme's assistant surgeon at the Royal Infirmary, so he discussed the idea with him. At first, Syme was surprised by Lister's request because the young surgeon was not licensed in Scotland and didn't have the experience usually required for such an advanced position. After thinking about the request, however, Syme agreed to his proposal because Lister was a skilled surgeon and scientifically curious. On April 21, 1854, Lister was elected a fellow of the Royal College of Surgeons in Scotland, allowing him to practice surgery in Edinburgh. Lister also began spending time with Syme at his home and met the family's older daughter.

Marriage

Lister was often a dinner guest at Syme's home and became interested in Agnes Symes, who was a plain girl blessed with a pleasant personality and keen intelligence.[173] Syme was not pleased about Lister's growing interest in his daughter because she was a member of the Episcopal Church of Scotland and Lister was a Quaker. Lister's parents also expressed concern about the marriage because of the couple's religious differences. He knew his love for Agnes was dangerous to his career, but Lister decided to marry her anyway. Lister realized he would have to give up his Quaker religion to marry Agnes, and he didn't know if his father would continue sending him money if he renounced the Quaker faith, but he didn't care because he loved Agnes. His father solved the issue by recommending Lister resign from the Quaker religion and assuring him of continued financial support even if he married Agnes.

Having reached an understanding with his father about religion and finances, Lister spoke to Symes, proposed to Agnes, and she accepted. Her mother set the wedding date for the following spring, and presents began rolling in. With Agnes's generous dowry and money from Lister's father, they bought a large home at 11 Rutledge Street, Edinburgh. The Georgian house had nine rooms on three floors, including a study off the main entrance that Lister converted to a consulting room where he saw patients. On April 23, 1856, they were married in Syme's drawing room out of consideration for Lister's family, who might have been uncomfortable attending a wedding in an Episcopal church.[174] After their honeymoon, Lister returned to studying hospital infections with Syme.

Research on Infections

When he returned to the Royal Infirmary, Lister faced the same problem—his surgical patients were dying from infections, and he didn't know how to prevent the deaths. Most surgeons believed they couldn't control whether their patients became infected following surgery, but Lister didn't agree that infections were inevitable. He continued taking samples of tissue from diseased patients to study under his microscope, hoping to understand what was happening when patients became infected. Lister wanted to understand what was causing inflammation and why some wounds became septic while others didn't. He noticed that when a bone fractured but didn't break the skin, the patient generally healed without getting infected while if a broken bone pierced the skin, infection often followed.[175] This suggested to Lister that something was entering the open wound from the air to make it septic, and he wanted to know how that happened and what he could do to prevent the infection.

Some surgeons believed infections were caused by chemicals or poisons in the air while other physicians argued that infections occurred by spontaneous generation, especially if the patient was in a weakened state as a result of an operation or old age. Everyone recognized that hospitals probably contributed to the incidence of infections, but no one knew why that happened or how to stop the infections. The level of hygiene that's routine in modern hospitals didn't exist in nineteenth-century operating rooms and hospital wards, and antibiotics would not be discovered for almost a century, so patients who were exposed to germs following surgery and contracted infections usually died. Lister wanted to change these septic hospital conditions and discover a way to prevent infections from spreading among his patients. While working on this problem with Syme in Edinburg, he was offered a position at the University of Glasgow.

University of Glasgow

In July 1859, James Lawrie, professor of clinical surgery at the University of Glasgow, suffered a stroke and had to resign. Lister was interested in the position but was concerned that if he moved to Glasgow, he would lose contact with Syme. He decided to apply for the position anyway, and Syme graciously sent a letter of recommendation to the University of Glasgow authorities supporting him. Lister heard nothing for months and assumed he had been rejected, but then learned he would be offered the post. However, local members of Parliament announced they wanted local physicians to vote on who should get the post, and Lister believed they would choose a Scotsman rather than him. However, leading Scottish surgeons protested Parliament's interference in their hiring process, and Lister was appointed to fill Lawrie's post at the University of Glasgow.[176]

Glasgow was a conservative university at the time and didn't welcome new ideas, so Lister was concerned about the impression he would make when he rose to give his acceptance speech. The speech had to be given in Latin, which was an unfamiliar language to Lister, but he soon settled into an easy rhythm and the Latin rolled off his tongue. After his opening remarks, the principal of the university rose and told him he had satisfied the first requirement of university appointment by proving he could speak Latin and could proceed in English. When he finished, Lister was welcomed as a professor of surgery at the University of Glasgow Medical School. Three hundred eleven students were accepted that year, and over half enrolled in Lister's surgery course. His lectures were a great success, and the students appreciated Lister's good humor. Once he was settled at the university, Lister applied for a position as the surgeon at Glasgow's Royal Infirmary because he wanted to demonstrate surgical methods to his students by operating on real patients.

The Royal Infirmary's board felt the hospital was for treatment, not education or medical research, and denied his request. All of Lister's medical students signed a letter saying they wanted him appointed to the position of surgeon at the Royal Infirmary so he could teach clinical surgery. Finally, in 1861, Lister was able to demonstrate surgical operations and lead medical students on surgical rounds in a new wing of the Royal Infirmary that accommodated six hundred patients. Lister was placed in charge of one female and two male wards. One male ward housed acute patients, and the other was reserved for chronic illnesses. Even though the hospital was new, diseases invaded the wards almost immediately. The acute ward was next to a graveyard where cholera patients had been buried during a recent outbreak, and that may have contributed to the spread of infections. Moreover, there were few provisions for washing hands or surgical instruments in the operating rooms, making infections likely.[177]

Although his patients were poor, Lister exhibited uncommon empathy for their comfort and well-being during and after surgery. He personally accompanied them from the operating room to the ward and helped make them comfortable. Once, when a little girl entered the hospital with a doll that had a limb torn off, Lister sewed the doll's severed limb back on and returned the toy to the little girl. She was delighted by his kindness and thanked him.

Lister published several articles on inflammation and designed new surgical instruments, but these accomplishments did little to cut the death rate from hospital infections, which was his primary goal. Lister decided to improve sanitation at the Royal Infirmary to see if he could reduce infections because he believed if the operating rooms and hospital wards were clean, there would be fewer deaths. He based this belief on reports by Alexander Gordon, a Scotsman; Oliver Wendell Holmes, Sr., an American; and Ignaz Semmelweis, an Austrian, who noted that women's wards under the care of medical students experienced significantly higher mortality rates compared with women's wards under the care of midwives.[178] They also reported that when medical students were required to wash their hands before attending patients in the maternity ward, mortality rates had fallen. Lister believed these reports supported his theory that small organisms had entered the open wounds and caused infections, which could be avoided by better sanitary conditions in hospital wards and operating rooms. He wanted to prove his idea experimentally but didn't know how to do that until he learned of Louis Pasteur's work on fermentation.

Pasteur's Theory

A chemistry professor named Thomas Anderson told Lister about Louis Pasteur's work on fermentation, and he became interested immediately.[179] English physicians had already learned that cholera was spread by contaminated water, which killed people who drank it when John Snow published his famous map showing deaths from cholera that were concentrated around the Broad Street water pump in London. When Snow persuaded authorities to remove the pump handle from the contaminated well, cholera disappeared in the area, supporting the idea that contaminated water was causing the cholera epidemic. But there were competing theories of what caused disease. Many physicians believed poisonous air caused disease. In 1858, when the banks of the Thames River became contaminated with human excrement and caused "the big stink," these physicians expected an epidemic would quickly follow. However, contrary to the poison-air theory of disease, no epidemic occurred, leading medical people to reject the idea that "bad air" caused disease. A few physicians began to believe small organisms might be causing infections by getting into open wounds, water, or the air people breathed. One of these physicians was Lister, and he wanted to apply Pasteur's theory to hospital infections.

Lister found a copy of Pasteur's publication in a bookstore and read it with interest. He learned that Pasteur's research began when a wine merchant told the French scientist that some of his vats turned sour during fermentation and he would like Pasteur to find out why that happened. At the time, scientists believed yeast was a catalyst for fermentation because they thought the conversion of sugar into alcohol was a chemical reaction, but Pasteur noticed that the sour wine vats smelled bad and were covered with an unusual film. He collected samples from the sour and sweet wine vats and studied them under his microscope. Pasteur found that the small organisms he observed in sour wine vats were different from the small organisms in normal vats of wine. The normal vats contained a small round organism while the sour vats contained a small elongated one. Pasteur speculated that the round organisms were causing fermentation and the elongated ones were souring the wine.

After extensive studies, Pasteur concluded that fermentation was a biological process and the yeast (round organism) that caused fermentation was a living organism rather than a catalyst.[180] He also concluded that yeast was not responsible for the spoiled wine, but instead, elongated bacteria had contaminated the sour vats and caused spoilage. Pasteur also hypothesized that yeasts and bacteria were present in the air and didn't spontaneously generate from inorganic matter. To test this hypothesis, Pasteur boiled grape juice to kill any microorganisms and placed the boiled juice in different-shaped containers. Some containers were ordinary flasks with an open top while others had S-shaped necks so dust and other particles from the air could not enter these flasks. Both sets of flasks were open to the air, but the flasks with S-shaped necks remained uncontaminated while the flasks with straight necks became contaminated with yeasts and other microbes. These results proved microbes such as yeasts and bacteria were present in the air because the flasks with the S-shaped necks would have become contaminated if organisms developed spontaneously, and they didn't. Pasteur concluded that only life begets life.

Lister was impressed with Pasteur's work and began his own series of experiments on fermentation to understand the process.[181] He accepted the idea that infections were caused by small organisms in the air, and these small microbes were causing fevers and death. Lister was beginning to formulate a theory that small organisms caused infections but didn't yet understand that different microbes can cause different diseases and small organisms could enter the body in several ways, such as drinking, breathing, or through an open wound. Lister believed he could not stop microbes from entering a wound because they were everywhere in the air according to Pasteur, so he set about trying to find a way to kill the microbes once they settled on a wound to prevent them from multiplying and causing an infection. He needed to find something that would kill harmful microbes before they multiplied and caused infection and death.

Antiseptic Surgery

Lister performed a series of experiments showing that the small creatures he saw in his microscope could be killed by heat, filtration, and chemicals. He knew that heat or filtration could not be used to sterilize wounds after surgery, so he began searching for a chemical that would kill microbes but not harm surrounding tissue. Antiseptics were already used following surgery if an infection occurred, but Lister believed by then it was too late. He studied several chemicals and found they were ineffective or damaged healthy tissue. Lister was having trouble finding a chemical that killed small organisms and was safe. He tried wine, quinine, iodine, and turpentine, but none proved effective and safe. Nitric acid had to be diluted to avoid harming tissue and then it didn't kill the microbes. Lister next tried potassium permanganate, but that didn't work either. He was running out of options but kept searching because he was determined to find a chemical that would safely kill the microbes.

One day, he recalled that engineers at sewage plants used carbolic acid to kill protozoa in sewage, so he decided to try that chemical as an antiseptic.[182] Carbolic acid is derived from coal tar and is poisonous at high concentrations, but Lister believed it might work if diluted with water, alcohol, olive oil, or another suitable liquid. In March of 1865, Lister excised a decaying bone in a patient's wrist and carefully washed the wound in dilute carbolic acid, but it still became infected. He was undeterred because he believed carbolic acid would work if he found the right concentration. Once he discovered the dilution of carbolic acid that killed microbes and didn't harm the surrounding tissue, Lister decided to test the antiseptic on compound fractures because microbes could only gain entrance through the wound itself rather than through other channels that might confuse the results of his study.

Treating Compound Fractures

Lister waited for compound fractures to come into the hospital so he could test carbolic acid as an antiseptic.[183] His first patient arrived in early August of 1865 when James Greenlees stepped into the street without looking and was run over by a cart. The wheel of the cart crushed his left leg, and the tibia was sticking through the skin. He arrived at the Royal Infirmary three hours later in critical condition because he had lost a lot of blood. Lister examined the leg and concluded the wound had been contaminated by small creatures from the wheel and while moving him to the infirmary, so he needed to operate and cleanse the wound. Acting quickly, Lister administered chloroform and began cleaning out the wound before microbes could multiply. He washed the wound with carbolic acid, covered it with putty so the acid would not be washed away by blood or lymph, and placed a tin lid over the wound to keep the carbolic acid from evaporating.

For three days, Lister carefully managed the wound, lifting the tin lid and pouring carbolic acid on the dressing to flush the wound every few hours. James's appetite returned after a few days, and Lister noted no rancid smell coming from the dressing. On the fourth day, Lister removed the dressing and saw that the skin was red around the wound, but not infected. The lack of pus was a good sign, but the inflammation bothered Lister. So he tried diluting the carbolic acid with water, but that didn't work. Next, he tried diluting carbolic acid with olive oil, and the inflammation around the wound disappeared. James Greenlees walked out of the Royal Infirmary on his own two legs thanks to the carbolic acid Lister used to sterilize his wound. Lister used carbolic acid on several other compound fractures, and most of them recovered without becoming infected. One patient died while Lister was on vacation, but the case had been supervised by another surgeon. Lister believed the other surgeon had not followed his instructions carefully. A second death was due to massive bleeding not noticed by the hospital staff until it was too late. Of the patients he treated with carbolic acid, eight avoided infections.[184] If he eliminated the patient cared for by another surgeon and the one that died of bleeding, Lister's cure rate using carbolic acid was over 90 percent.

Before he published his results, Lister wanted to prove carbolic acid could prevent infections in patients coming directly from the operating room because if carbolic acid worked under those conditions, more complex surgeries could be performed and more patients might live. Additional studies showed that carbolic acid could sterilize wounds from an operation, so Lister began publishing his research in *The Lancet* on March 16, 1867. In a series of articles, Lister reported he had developed a sterilization system based on Pasteur's theory that putrefaction was caused by microbes in the air and wrote that it was necessary to sterilize the wound with a chemical capable of killing microbes before it became infected. Lister said he had used dilute carbolic acid to kill small organisms on the wound and it worked.[185] His papers presented case studies intended to teach readers how to use his antiseptic methods to prevent infection. Lister was about to face a personal test of his sterilization technique when his sister entered his office with a medical problem.

Breast Cancer

His sister, Isabella Pim, arrived at Lister's home in Glasgow and announced that she had discovered a lump in her breast and was concerned it might be cancer. After examining her, Lister agreed she had cancer and recommended a mastectomy. He went to the dissecting room at the university and performed the operation on a cadaver for practice. He also discussed her case with Syme, and they agreed an operation would give her the best chance to survive. On June 16, 1867, Isabella entered her brother's temporary operating room in his home to prepare for the operation. Lister soaked his instruments in carbolic acid and administered chloroform to induce deep sleep in his sister. He dipped his hands in carbolic acid, cleaned the site of the operation, and carefully removed the affected breast, muscles, and lymph nodes. He then covered her chest with gauze soaked in carbolic acid and covered the gauze with a cotton cloth soaked in the antiseptic. Layers of gauze and cotton allowed the wound to discharge without the carbolic acid evaporating or being washed from the wound.

Her wound healed without infection because of Lister's careful application of carbolic acid–soaked gauze and cotton, and his sister lived three more years before cancer appeared in her liver. Lister gave a lecture describing the operation to the British Medical Association on August 9, 1867, entitled "On the Antiseptic Principle in the Practice of Surgery." Shortly after his lecture to the British Medical Association, the editor of *The Lancet* expressed cautious support for Lister's antiseptic method. Meanwhile, Lister learned that Syme had suffered a stroke and lost use of the left side of his body, so he and Agnes returned to Edinburgh to care for him. Syme resigned from the university and recommended Lister as his replacement. On August 18, 1869, Lister was offered the chair of clinical surgery at the University of Edinburgh and he accepted. He and Agnes moved to Edinburg to care for Syme and begin his new job. In June of 1870, Syme died after losing the ability to speak. While this was happening, conservative surgeons began expressing doubts about Lister's work.

Criticisms of Lister

Conservative older surgeons rejected Lister's theory about microbes and believed his postoperative treatments were too complicated and not necessary. One surgeon stated that treating an infected wound with carbolic acid helped, but he did not believe washing a wound with carbolic acid would prevent infections. Many surgeons who tried Lister's methods didn't follow his instructions; their patients became infected, and they rejected his theory that carbolic acid could prevent infections caused by microbes in the air. Most older surgeons were unwilling to believe invisible organisms could cause disease and rejected Lister's theory.[186] Undeterred, Lister believed his best tactic was to train a new generation of medical students on antiseptic methods, so he lectured on theories of infection and presented case studies and demonstrations of his sterilization method to young medical students and surgeons. He also replied to critics who claimed that the mortality rate in the Glasgow Royal Infirmary had not changed after he introduced antiseptic procedures.

Lister collected death rates at the Royal Infirmary for 1864–66 (before he introduced carbolic acid sterilization) and for 1867–68 (after he introduced his sterile procedures). His results showed that the mortality rate had dropped from 46 percent to 15 percent due to the use of carbolic acid—a significant improvement.[187] Lister's paper prompted the editors of *The Lancet* to recommend that physicians and surgeons test Lister's methods for themselves and that Lister's students be allowed to supervise the tests so that they were done properly and would be fair. In 1871, Lister was asked to attend Queen Victoria, who had become seriously ill.

Queen Victoria

Lister arrived by carriage at Balmoral Castle, the Scottish home of Queen Victoria, in response to a telegram requesting he visit her. The queen had developed an abscess in her armpit that grew to about six inches in diameter, and her physicians recommended she call a surgeon to have the abscess removed. Lister brought his medical equipment and a new carbolic acid spray machine intended to remove harmful microbes from the air during an operation and when changing dressings. He examined the queen and told her he needed to operate immediately. She gave permission, and he decided to administer a mild dose of chloroform because of the queen's weak condition. Lister disinfected his hands, instruments, and the area under the queen's arm while his assistant filled the air with carbolic acid spray during the procedure. He made an incision in the queen's armpit, and blood and pus gushed from the abscess. Lister cleaned the wound and bandaged it with a carbolic acid–soaked cloth. The next morning, he noticed that pus had formed under the bandage; so he took a rubber tube off the atomizer, washed it in carbolic acid, and inserted the tube into the queen's wound to drain off the pus. The next day, clear lymph was flowing from the wound, and Lister was relieved.[188] His surgical technique, antiseptic procedure, and quick thinking to drain the wound saved Queen Victoria's life. News of his successful treatment of the queen spread, confirming the efficacy of his antiseptic methods and increasing Lister's fame.

Lister's classes overflowed with medical students after his successful treatment of Queen Victoria, and he traveled the world discussing the benefits of antiseptic surgery. The Lancet's call to test Lister's theory had worked, and more surgeons were convinced that antiseptic surgery helped avoid infections. Doctors in Glasgow and Edinburgh were ahead of London physicians in applying Lister's antiseptic techniques, but hospital conditions in America were worse; Lister's antiseptic techniques were banned in major American hospitals because they were believed to be too complicated and not effective. Lister decided to visit America and try to convince physicians and surgeons they should try using antiseptics when doing surgery. He was scheduled to speak at the International Medical Congress in Philadelphia and planned to present his antiseptic techniques and case studies to American physicians at that time.

Lister in America

On September 4, 1876, Lister entered the chapel at the University of Pennsylvania to attend the International Medical Congress. His ideas about disease and antiseptics were criticized by several American doctors who claimed there was no proof that microbes cause illness. On the second day of the Congress, Lister made his way to the front of the chapel to present a defense of his antiseptic methods. He began by giving credit to William Morton, the American doctor and dentist who had introduced anesthesia for use during surgery, and then Lister discussed the benefits of antiseptic surgery, pointing out the relation between microbes, infection, and pus. He outlined several case studies and concluded that if the microbes are destroyed during and after surgery, no pus will form and the patient would be free of infection. His presentation was rejected by a hostile audience convinced that Lister was wrong.

Undeterred, Lister set out on a speaking tour to San Francisco and back to the East Coast.[189] He taught groups of doctors and medical students about his antiseptic technique, and surgeons who tested his theory on patients became supporters of Lister's work. In New York City, Lister performed an operation attended by over one hundred medical students. He began the operation in his usual way by washing his hands, his instruments, the operating table, and the patient with carbolic acid and had it sprayed in the air during the procedure. Lister told his audience they needed to rigorously apply the antiseptic method before, during, and after the operation to safeguard the patient's health. He drained pus from the patient's wound, washed it with carbolic acid, and applied an antiseptic dressing. When the demonstration was complete, the audience of medical students rose and cheered. His biggest American triumph happened in Boston, however.

Lister was invited to speak at Harvard University when he returned to the East Coast and was welcomed by young medical students. After the lecture, the director of Massachusetts General Hospital, Dr. Henry Bigelow, endorsed Lister's antiseptic technique; and Massachusetts General became the first medical institution in America to approve his antiseptic technique, an astonishing turnaround for the American hospital that had banned antiseptic techniques and threatened to fire any surgeon who used the procedure before Lister gave his lecture.[190] When he returned to the United Kingdom, Lister was presented with a new opportunity.

King's College London

Soon after he returned to Scotland, King's College London offered him a position as a professor of surgery. Lister was interested but said he needed a guarantee of total freedom in the classroom and hospital before he would accept the post. The college reluctantly accepted his conditions, and he left Edinburg for London in 1877. Lister felt confident that his Scottish medical students would maintain clean wards, antiseptic conditions, and good ventilation in Edinburg hospitals as he had taught them. Years later, he went to Paris to celebrate Louis Pasteur's life, work, and birthday.

In 1892, Lister traveled to Paris to attend a celebration of Louis Pasteur's seventieth birthday. They entered the Sorbonne together, both important men who were nearing the end of their professional lives. Pasteur was not in good health because he had suffered a stroke. Lister gave Pasteur credit for suggesting the idea of antiseptic surgery, and the auditorium erupted in applause at his generous gesture. Pasteur embraced his friend for the last time because they would never meet again. When he returned to England, Lister was knighted and elected president of the Royal Society at the International Medical Congress in London for his work on antiseptic surgery.[191] Quite a change from earlier years when his ideas had been rejected in England and America. He was also appointed personal surgeon to Queen Victoria and awarded honorary doctorates from Oxford and Cambridge universities.

Lister died on February 11, 1912, at the age of eighty-four in his country home.[192] By his bed was an unfinished paper discussing the nature and causes of suppuration (the formation, conversion, or discharge of pus from an abscess). He worked until the end of his life trying to save patients from unnecessary death. A public funeral was held at Westminster Abbey, and he was buried at Hampstead Cemetery, London, in the central chapel. There is a marble medallion of Lister in Westminster Abbey next to medallions of Darwin, Stokes, Adams, and Watt, all famous English men of science.

Chapter 9

Chapter 9

- - - - ⚜ - - - -

GERM THEORY: ROBERT KOCH

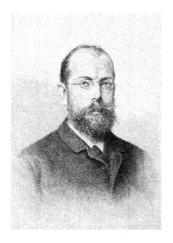

R obert Koch was impressed by Pasteur's work on fermentation and microbes and set out to learn what caused anthrax after a local farmer reported that his sheep were dying. Koch collected blood from a dead sheep, examined it under his microscope, and saw small rods and threads in the dead sheep's blood. He found that the rods and threads were always present in the blood of sick or dead sheep, but never appeared in the blood of healthy animals. Koch grew the small rods and threads in a test tube and found they died when exposed to sunlight. He wondered how anthrax was able to survive from one year to the next in a pasture if the rods and threads died when exposed to sunlight in his laboratory. One day, when he looked at a slide containing anthrax rods and threads, Koch saw they had turned into spores. He realized anthrax could survive exposure to sunlight in a pasture because the rods and threads had developed a protective coating. Next, he collected tissue from a laborer who died of tuberculosis and studied it under his microscope but saw nothing. Koch decided to try staining the infected tissue and discovered that methylene blue dye allowed him to see tuberculosis bacilli. Koch's theory of germs helped millions of people avoid contracting contagious diseases.

Koch was born on December 11, 1843, in Clausthal, Prussia. His father was an engineer, director of a mining company, and mining adviser to the Prussian government. By the time he was five, Koch was reading the local newspaper. He considered following his older brother to America but wanted to get an education first and then decide on his future. Koch graduated from Clausthal Gymnasium in 1862, where he learned Latin, Greek, French, and English. When the Koch family inherited some property, Koch's father enrolled him in Gottingen University to study mathematics, physics, and botany.[193]

Gottingen University

A few months after he arrived at Gottingen University, Koch decided he wanted to study medicine rather than physics and become an army physician so he could travel to exotic foreign lands. As a physician, he made major contributions to the field of bacteriology and proved that germs cause infections.[194] At medical school, he worked with the famous anatomist Jacob Henle, who had recently published a book on contagious diseases that Koch read with interest. When Koch was in medical school, no one understood that bacteria cause disease, and infections can occur by touching a contaminated surface, breathing bacteria from the air, drinking infected water, or by germs entering an open wound. Germ theory had little scientific support before Koch began his work on the relationship between bacteria and diseases.

Koch was appointed assistant in the Museum of Pathology while he was still in medical school. His doctoral thesis explored the origin of butyric acid in humans (a fatty acid created in the human gut by bacteria).[195] Koch tried to be his own subject by eating a pound of butter a day, which contains large quantities of butyric acid but decided to use animals in his research after he fell ill from the diet. He graduated with honors in 1866, moved to Berlin for his internship, and began studying infectious diseases.

Berlin

Koch served his medical internship at the Charity Hospital in Berlin and was unhappy about the hospital conditions he found. Patients were crowded into small rooms, and interns didn't have a clear view of what their anatomy professor was trying to demonstrate during a dissection. Koch wanted a commission as an army doctor so he could travel the world, but Europe was at peace and all the army medical commissions were filled.[196] Since there was no chance for him to enter the army as a physician, Koch decided to become a ship's doctor on a passenger liner as an alternative so he could travel. He wrote to his family about the idea, but his mother didn't want her son to leave Germany and decided to take matters into her own hands by contacting the girl Robert had been seeing to let her know his plans. Emmy Josephine Fraatz decided to meet Koch when he returned home for vacation and discuss their future.

Engagement to Emmy

When confronted by his mother and Emmy, Koch quickly changed his mind about becoming a ship's doctor and announced his engagement to Emmy.[197] Back in Berlin, Koch was offered an assistantship in the General Hospital at Hamburg after he passed the state medical examination, and he accepted. Koch finished his internship, passed the examination, and traveled to Hamburg to begin his new career working at the city's general hospital. Soon after Koch settled in Hamburg, he began doing research on contagious diseases after the city experienced an epidemic of cholera. The disease was common in large international ports because ships brought many infectious diseases from Asia. Little was known about cholera in 1866, and there was no vaccine for the disease when Koch began his research.

Studying Cholera

Cholera was thought to be transmitted by unsanitary food and water, but no one was certain what actually caused the illness. Symptoms included diarrhea, vomiting, weakness, and death.[198] Koch was excited to have the opportunity to study the disease among his hospital patients and set about collecting tissue samples from cholera patients to study under his microscope. He made drawings of the microbes he saw in the diseased tissue but was too inexperienced to understand that he was actually seeing the bacteria that caused cholera. Years later, after he had studied anthrax and tuberculosis, Koch was able to recognize cholera bacilli when he saw them under his microscope, but when he first began studying infectious diseases, he didn't know for certain that bacteria were causing contagious diseases.

While Koch was beginning his research on cholera, Emmy persuaded his uncle to invite her to Hamburg so she could see Robert.[199] While walking along Hamburg Harbor together, Koch told Emmy he would like to travel to distant lands and asked if she was interested in joining him. She replied, "If you love me, you must stay here at home." Koch immediately realized he had a serious decision to make—stay and marry Emmy or leave her and see faraway lands. After thinking about his options, he decided to marry Emmy and told her he planned to develop a medical practice in Germany and that they would be married soon. To fulfill his promise to Emmy, Koch resigned from the general hospital in Hamburg, took a position as an assistant physician in a mental hospital near Hanover, and opened a private medical practice. His medical practice prospered, and Koch was soon making enough money to marry Emmy. On July 16, 1867, they were married in Clausthal.[200] Emmy's father performed the ceremony in his own church.

Due to financial problems at the mental hospital in Langenhagen, Koch was told they no longer had a position for him as an assistant physician, so he began looking for another city where he could practice medicine and study bacteria with his microscope. He settled in Niemegk, near Potsdam, but found the villagers preferred home remedies rather than the scientific medicine Koch practiced; so he moved to Rakwitz, a town near the Polish border with Germany. Koch soon discovered he needed an interpreter to understand some of his patients because many spoke only Polish. At first, his practice grew slowly; but after Koch treated a wealthy citizen who had wounded himself with a revolver, word spread that Dr. Koch was a fine physician, and his practice flourished. He was happy during this period, especially when his daughter Gertrude was born.[201] Koch enjoyed a comfortable homelife, a thriving medical practice, and had time to work with his microscope studying infectious diseases. However, war was declared between Germany and France, and he was called to army service.

Army Surgeon

In 1870, soon after war broke out between Germany and France, Koch joined the army as a physician. Well-trained German troops crossed the French border, and General von Moltke won a decisive victory over the French at Sedan in September of 1870. Koch was assigned to a field hospital as a surgeon and was shocked by the casualties he encountered during the war. However, he didn't get to travel to foreign lands; Koch was assigned to a military hospital at Neufchâteau where he treated soldiers who had contracted typhoid fever. Koch diagnosed and treated typhoid patients, and his experience with this infectious disease proved invaluable in his later studies of germs.[202] The Franco-Prussian War was nearly over when the village of Rakwitz begged the German government to release "Herr Doctor Koch" so he could come home and treat them. Koch was released from the army and given a hero's welcome when he returned to Rakwitz. A few months after he returned from the army, Koch applied for the post of district physician in Wollstein, a town near Posen. He took the required examination, passed, and was offered the job. Now he had a steady salary, a private medical practice, and time to study bacteria and disease with his microscope.

Wollstein

Koch spent eight fruitful years in Wollstein studying infectious diseases and pioneering the field of bacteriology, the study of how microbes cause illnesses.[203] He was a fine physician, and many patients from around the area came to him for treatment. Koch kept guinea pigs, monkeys, mice, pigeons, dogs, cats, and even a fox for use in his experiments on infectious diseases. He quickly settled into the life of a busy country doctor, but never gave up his passion for studying bacteria with a microscope. Koch established a small laboratory in his medical office, separated by a curtain from the remainder of his consulting room. He also had a darkroom built so he could develop photographs of interesting bacteria he saw in his microscope.[204] Koch had Emmy watch the sky and tell him when the sun was out so he could photograph an important bacterial specimen in good light through his microscope. He read Louis Pasteur's work on fermentation and microbes; became excited by the idea that bacteria are everywhere in the air, water, and food; and set out to find the germs that cause diseases. Koch began to collect bits of tissue from infected patients for study under the microscope and found he needed to keep his slides clean so they didn't become contaminated. He made his first important discovery of germs when he began studying what was killing sheep in the area around his medical practice.

Anthrax

In 1876, Koch made an important finding concerning the cause of infectious disease when a local farmer reported that his sheep were dying. Koch went to examine the dying sheep and found that some were healthy, some were dead, and others were too sick to eat. He carefully drew blood from a dead sheep and discovered it was black rather than red as normal blood should be. Koch placed the black blood in a vial, returned home, and spread blood from the dead sheep on a slide to study under his microscope. What he saw confirmed his ideas about the cause of infectious disease—he observed thin rods and threads in the black blood of the dead sheep.[205] Koch concluded that the microbes he was seeing were killing the animals and set out to prove his theory was correct.

Koch studied samples of blood from several sheep killed by anthrax and found rods and threads in every blood sample from the infected animals. The little rods and threads were always present in diseased sheep, but Koch could never find rods or threads in the blood of healthy sheep. He believed he had discovered the microbe that was causing anthrax. Koch knew that finding a cure for anthrax was important because animals could be healthy in the morning, become sick, and die the next day from being infected with anthrax. More than likely, the farmer who tended the infected sheep would also catch the disease and die from a fit of coughing a few days later. The fatality rate of inhaled anthrax was nearly 80 percent among humans.[206]

Studies of Anthrax

Others had also seen tiny rods and threads through their microscopes but had not understood that the microbes were causing anthrax. Koch studied hundreds of samples of blood from diseased and healthy animals and concluded that Pasteur was right—microbes cause disease. He believed the rods and threads seen in his microscope were causing anthrax and decided to grow the small rods and threads in a test tube so he could study them before publishing his conclusions. Koch began to formulate a plan for how to grow anthrax in a test tube and decided the first step was to infect white mice with anthrax germs and see what happened. To infect his mice with anthrax, Koch used a wood sliver that he cleaned and passed through a flame to kill any existing bacteria. He made a tiny cut in the tail of a mouse, dipped the sterilized sliver of wood in blood from an animal that had died of anthrax, and inserted some of the diseased blood into the cut on the mouse's tail.

Koch infected a healthy mouse with anthrax using this method, placed it in a cage, and put the infected animal aside to see what happened. He took care of patients and went to bed wondering what he would see the next day. In the morning, Koch found that the infected white mouse was dead. When he dissected the animal, Koch found that the spleen was black and swollen. He believed the mouse had died of anthrax; so Koch took a bit of tissue from the animal's spleen, placed it under his microscope, and saw the same tiny anthrax rods and threads he had observed before, indicating he had successfully infected the mouse with anthrax. He took blood from the dead mouse and infected a healthy mouse to verify his conclusion. The newly infected mouse died in twenty-four hours. Koch repeated the experiment thirty times, and all thirty mice died within twenty-four hours from anthrax infection.[207] He extracted blood from each of the dead mice and observed the same tiny rods and threads of anthrax bacilli in the diseased-mouse blood that he had seen in dead-sheep blood.

Growing Anthrax in a Test Tube

Koch next wanted to see if he could grow anthrax rods and threads in a test tube, but he needed a way to feed the bacteria. He tried several media for growing anthrax in a test tube before he discovered that a hollowed-out well in a glass slide, heated beforehand to kill any bacteria, and filled with a drop of serum from the eye of an ox, worked fine for growing anthrax. Koch sealed the ox-eye serum in the slide well by spreading petroleum jelly around the well and placing a second glass slide on top of the serum and anthrax bacilli. The anthrax rods and threads were protected from contamination, and because the apparatus was glass, Koch could observe through his microscope what was happening within the drop of ox-eye fluid that contained the anthrax microbes.

When he first placed the glass slide containing anthrax bacilli and ox serum under his microscope, Koch saw nothing for a few hours. Then he began to see tiny rods and threads grow and divide in the ox-eye fluid. Within a few hours, Koch's tiny drop of infected ox-eye serum was filled with anthrax rods and threads. He repeated the experiment with infected drops of ox-eye serum eight times and saw the same thing every time—thousands of small rods and threads growing and dividing in the ox-eye serum as he looked at the slide under his microscope. Next, he injected some of the anthrax bacilli from his ox-eye serum into a healthy mouse to see if anthrax bacilli grown in a test tube would infect and kill the healthy animal. Twenty-four hours later, the infected mouse was dead. When he dissected the dead mouse and took a piece of infected spleen tissue for study, he saw anthrax rods and threads with his microscope. Koch injected serum containing anthrax grown in a test tube into other healthy animals, including sheep, guinea pigs, rabbits, and cats. Each time, the animal died, and Koch was able to observe anthrax bacilli in the blood or tissue of the dead animal under his microscope.

Anthrax Spores

Next, Koch wanted to find a way to kill anthrax bacilli so he could advise farmers on how to save their flocks. He noticed that sometimes anthrax bacilli failed to grow in the ox-eye fluid and wondered why. After extensive investigation, Koch noticed that when anthrax rods and threads were exposed to sunlight, they died.[208] He was confused. How could anthrax bacilli infect sheep in a pasture after being exposed to sunshine for months, but die in his laboratory when exposed to sunlight? Koch wondered how anthrax rods and threads survived from one year to the next in pastures but died when exposed to sunlight in his laboratory. He couldn't understand how the disease could survive in a pasture where it was exposed to sunlight for months at a time.

Koch found the answer one day when he looked at a glass slide containing anthrax bacilli, expecting to see rods and threads in the ox-eye fluid, but instead observed tiny oval objects that looked like beads strung together like a pearl necklace. At first, he wondered if the beads were another microbe that had somehow contaminated his slide, but after carefully repeating the procedure several times, Koch concluded that the beads had developed from the rods and threads of anthrax bacilli he had placed on the slide for examination. He dried the specimen of anthrax containing the small beads and put it away to examine later. After a few weeks, Koch decided to see what would happen if he placed some of the anthrax beads in ox-eye serum. He found that the beads grew into anthrax rods and threads and concluded that the beads were *spores* that allowed anthrax to survive outside in sunlight over the winter and infect animals the next spring.[209]

Koch also placed ox-eye serum contaminated with anthrax bacilli on ice and saw that the rods and threads didn't grow when they were cold. He now knew what advice to give the farmers about anthrax: bury all dead animals so the anthrax bacilli could not form spores and spread into the pasture to infect animals the next year. Koch had discovered the life cycle of anthrax bacilli and wanted to share his discovery with science and farmers. He wrote a letter to Dr. Ferdinand Cohn of the Botanical Institute in Breslau describing his work with anthrax bacilli. Dr. Cohn invited Koch to come to Breslau and demonstrate his discoveries to a group of medical experts.

Breslau Report on Anthrax

On April 30, 1876, Dr. Cohn invited physiologists, pathologists, and an expert on staining tissues to attend Koch's lecture. As Koch proceeded, the experts began to pay close attention. He began by growing a pure strain of anthrax bacilli in a test tube, staining the bacilli with Weigert's dyes, and showing how the anthrax bacilli develop from spores in ox-eye serum.[210] He also injected anthrax bacilli grown in a test tube into mice to show they killed healthy animals. Koch repeated his demonstrations several times to prove the anthrax bacillus retained its lethality outside an animal either in a test tube or as spores and caused a deadly anthrax infection when injected into healthy mice.

The medical experts were impressed and invited their students to see Dr. Koch's work. He explained that he believed only anthrax bacilli cause anthrax and only typhoid bacilli cause typhoid. Members of the audience shook Koch's hand and congratulated him when he was finished. They suggested Koch submit his work to Rudolf Virchow, the most famous German medical scientist at the time. However, Virchow didn't seem to understand what Koch had discovered, so he decided to draft an article and publish it in a medical journal. Koch sent the forty-page article to Dr. Cohn, who published it in *Contributions to the Biology of Plants*. Today, the article is considered a classic in the history of bacteriology. Koch also published a paper describing how to stain microbes so they could be photographed more clearly and another describing his theory of germs and disease.

Koch's Germ Theory

In 1878, Koch published an article describing his investigations of wound infections and criticized scientists who believed microbes could transform themselves from one type of bacillus into another. Koch argued that every microbe has its own shape and causes a unique disease. Based on his work with anthrax, Koch was appointed city physician of Breslau in 1880, which allowed him to spend more time working on infectious diseases. A few months later, the German government offered him the post at the Imperial Health Office in Berlin, and Koch accepted because he would be able to work full-time on research while employed by the city.[211]

When he arrived in Berlin, Koch found a well-equipped laboratory waiting for him with all the materials he needed for his work. If he required a piece of special equipment, there were funds to buy or manufacture it. Koch was also assigned two bright young military doctors as research assistants. At first, he didn't know what to do with the assistants because he was used to doing everything himself. Soon they were working as a team. Koch needed pure cultures of microbes in his research, so he and his assistants set out to separate one microbe from a mix of several. They tried several techniques for separating bacteria, but nothing seemed to work.

Pure Germ Cultures

Then one morning when he entered the laboratory, Koch noticed that a slice of boiled potato left on a table had developed tiny spots overnight, and the spots were of different colors—some red, others yellow or violet. Using a piece of thin wire, Koch transferred material from one of the colored spots to a glass slide and looked at it under his microscope. He was not surprised to see thousands of microbes, but he was astonished when he realized they were all alike! The potato spot contained a pure culture of a single microbe.[212] Koch examined material from other spots on the potato and found that each contained one type of microbe. Some were rods, others corkscrews, and still others round organisms, but each sample from a single spot on the boiled potato was a pure culture of a single bacillus. Koch showed the pure cultures to his assistants, who were equally surprised. They asked how Koch had developed them, and he replied that nature had done it for him and they now had a procedure for growing pure cultures in the laboratory. After thinking about the process, Koch developed a theory of how single bacterial cultures grow.

Koch speculated that when microbes fall from the air into a liquid medium, they mix with other microbes; but when a germ falls on a solid medium, it has to stay in that one spot and grow. By growing microbes in a single spot on a solid medium, Koch believed he could collect and grow pure cultures. Koch and his assistants went to work testing his theory by spreading various microbes on the sides of boiled potatoes and discovered that wherever a unique microbe landed on the potato, it stayed in that spot and multiplied as a pure colony. They next tried to develop a solid medium for growing pure microbes in the laboratory. Koch found that warm liquid gelatin mixed with beef broth and poured in large shallow dishes worked quite well after it had cooled. When the mixtures solidified, Koch set the shallow dishes aside to see if microbes settled on the surface and grew into single pure colonies of bacteria. Later, when he looked in his microscope, he saw single cultures of microbes, showing he had found a method of growing pure cultures in the laboratory. Koch then established a set of rules to guide his work that became the guiding principles of bacteriology.

Koch's Rules

His rules are as follows:

1.   To prove that a microbe causes a disease, you must find the microbe in every case of the disease but not in healthy animals.
2.   The microbe must be separated from the diseased body and grown in a test tube as a pure culture.

3. The pure culture grown in a test tube must produce the disease when injected into a healthy animal.

4. The same microbe should then be extracted from the new diseased animal and grown as a pure culture outside the body.

Once he had formulated his rules, Koch began studying tuberculosis.

Tuberculosis

In August of 1881, the Imperial Health Ministry sent Koch to the International Medical Congress in London, where he met Louis Pasteur and Joseph Lister. Koch was planning to study tuberculosis, and he talked with everyone about the disease. During the nineteenth century, one out of every seven people who became infected with tuberculosis died. Koch wanted to find out what caused the disease and how to cure it. In 1839, Dr. J. L. Schoenbein found tiny lumps that he called tubercles in the bodies of persons who had died from tuberculosis. Physicians knew tuberculosis was caused by a microbe because they were able to transmit the disease from an infected human to an animal, but they had no idea what germ was causing the illness. Scientists searched for the tuberculosis germ, but no one was able to see the microbe because it was too small to be visible using existing microscopes.[213]

In 1881, he collected samples of tissue from a laborer who had died of tuberculosis and studied the infected tissue under his microscope. Koch could see nothing. He infected guinea pigs and rabbits with tissue from dead tuberculosis patients, watched the animals die, and still could not see the microbe in his microscope. He decided tuberculosis was too small to see unless he stained it with the proper dye. Koch tried different methods of staining the germ before he prepared a specimen of tuberculosis tissue using methylene blue dye. He then saw tuberculosis bacilli for the first time.[214] They were much smaller than anthrax, but visible in his microscope when dyed. He saw tiny blue curved rods in the tissue of tuberculosis patients but was not able to find such crescent rods in tissue from healthy humans.

Koch next took samples from rabbits he had infected with tuberculosis, stained the tissue with methylene blue, and placed them under his microscope. He found the same little curved blue rods. Koch now needed to show that the same tuberculosis bacillus appeared in every case of the disease but not in tissue from healthy patients. He asked every hospital in Berlin to send him tissue samples from tuberculosis patients. Koch used diseased tissue from humans who had died from tuberculosis to infect hundreds of mice, dogs, pigs, cats, and chickens. Some of the animals infected with tuberculosis died, and when he stained the infected tissue from the dead animals and studied it under a microscope, Koch always found the blue crescent rods. His assistants urged him to publish, but Koch said he wanted to grow a pure culture of the tuberculosis microbe in a test tube and infect animals with it before he published.

Culturing Tuberculosis

Koch tried to grow tuberculosis bacillus in beef broth and gelatin soups at different temperatures, but none of his mixtures worked. He decided to duplicate conditions inside a human body by using blood serum jelly warmed in an incubator. Koch collected blood serum from butcher shops, filled several test tubes with the serum, heated it to kill any existing microbes, and when it hardened, he placed tuberculosis tissue from a dead guinea pig on the solid blood serum surface. Koch placed the tubes filled with infected serum in an incubator set at the body temperature of a rabbit and waited.

Two weeks later, he was getting discouraged because nothing had happened. He considered throwing out the tubes but decided to take one more look through his microscope. Koch stained the blood serum with methylene blue dye, looked at it under the microscope, and saw small blue crescent rods characteristic of tuberculosis.[215] He repeated the experiment forty times to make certain his procedure was reliable. Next, Koch infected healthy animals with tuberculosis bacilli grown in a test tube to make certain it caused disease in living animals. He infected turtles, fish, dogs, rabbits, and cats with the test-tube-grown tuberculosis bacilli. Weeks later, the fish and turtles were healthy, but some of the mammals were dying. Koch examined tissue from each dead mammal under his microscope and found blue crescent rods of tuberculosis bacilli when he stained the tissue. He had completed the four steps of his procedure and now knew the cause of tuberculosis.

On March 24, 1882, Koch presented his findings on tuberculosis to the Berlin Physiological Society. The most famous men in German science were there to hear Koch. After his clear and careful presentation, there was no discussion or questions for the first time in the society's history. Everyone agreed that Koch had done an extraordinary job of showing the cause of tuberculosis, and there was no question unanswered. Two weeks later, he published his famous paper titled "The Etiology of Tuberculosis" in the *Berlin Clinical Weekly*.[216] Doctors around the world began following Koch's directions and staining tuberculosis bacilli for themselves to confirm his results. Koch was now famous, and young doctors from around the world came to study in his laboratory. He also proved tuberculosis bacilli could infect an animal through the air by spraying tuberculosis bacilli from a dead animal into a box that contained healthy animals. All the animals in the box contracted tuberculosis. Koch next decided to study cholera to discover what microbe causes that dread disease.

Cholera

In the summer of 1883, cholera broke out in Egypt and was threatening Europe. Originally from India, the disease had spread throughout the world, and Europeans were terrified because people feared it would be brought to European ports by a ship. The Egyptian government asked France and Germany for help to combat the disease by sending experts to study its cause. Koch went to Egypt as the leading expert on infectious disease. He examined the bodies of hundreds of cholera victims and injected tissue from the victims into animals, hoping to infect them with the disease, but nothing happened. Then cholera mysteriously disappeared from Egypt. He was determined to continue his work but needed an active source of cholera.

Koch asked the German government if he could go to India to study cholera and was given permission.[217] He left for Calcutta in December 1883 where he studied patients with cholera and found bacilli in the intestines of sick patients. Koch could not find the cholera bacillus in healthy patients' intestines; and he believed that tiny crescent-shaped germs, fatter than tuberculosis bacilli, were the cause of cholera. He called them *comma bacilli* and found that they grew in beef-broth jelly or blood serum. Koch also found that cholera bacilli died when heated. He found cholera microbes in well water in the city of Calcutta and decided that was probably how cholera spread.[218] He believed cholera victims were drinking contaminated water, contracting the disease, and spreading it through clothes and bedsheets to others.

Koch concluded that poor sanitation spreads cholera in water, food, and clothing. He thought unsanitary conditions on ships likely transported cholera from India to Egypt and Europe. He suggested using strong disinfectants such as carbolic acid to suppress the disease on ships. When he returned home, Koch was awarded the Order of the Crown by Kaiser Wilhelm of Germany, who also gave him one hundred thousand marks for his discovery of the cholera bacillus. He reported to the German medical community that cholera is caused by comma bacillus, grows in the human gut, and is contracted by drinking polluted water or eating contaminated food. Koch began looking for a way to treat tuberculosis after he returned to Berlin.

Tuberculin Test

Koch accepted a professorship at the University of Berlin and became head of the Hygiene Institute when he returned from India. He gave a course on the diagnosis and treatment of cholera, and doctors from around the world came to study in his laboratory.[219] Koch began working on a cure after he noticed that guinea pigs injected with tuberculosis developed an ulcer that did not go away where he had made the injection. However, if he injected a second dose of the tuberculosis bacilli in the same animal, the injection site healed. He wondered if the second dose of tuberculosis bacilli was acting as a vaccine. Koch tried infecting guinea pigs who were just beginning to develop tuberculosis with a second dose of the disease, and their health improved. Had he found a vaccine for tuberculosis?

Koch wondered if an injection of sterile dead tuberculosis bacilli would give animals immunity to the disease. He called the sterile liquid *tuberculin* and began planning a series of studies to confirm he could inoculate animals and humans against tuberculosis.[220] Koch was pressured by German authorities to announce his discovery at the Tenth International Medical Conference in Berlin before he completed his work. He agreed to announce his work on tuberculin at the Berlin conference but was careful to say his results were preliminary. He did report he had stopped the growth of tuberculosis in animals and concluded his presentation by saying that guinea pigs, who are especially susceptible to tuberculosis, no longer caught tuberculosis after being treated with tuberculin. The press announced that Koch had found a cure for tuberculosis, which was premature and turned out to be wrong.

Koch clarified his conclusions soon after the conference, saying tuberculin did not help those with advanced tuberculosis. He had hoped tuberculin would be an effective vaccine against tuberculosis, but it didn't work. Today, tuberculin is used as a test for diagnosing exposure to tuberculosis.[221] The modern test uses a patch soaked with tuberculin and attached to a person's skin for a few days. If the person has been exposed to tuberculosis in the past, redness and swelling appear where the patch was applied, but nothing happens if the person has not been exposed to tuberculosis. When antibiotics were discovered in the early twentieth century, tuberculosis could finally be cured although some variants have become resistant to many modern antibiotics. In 1960, a vaccine was developed for tuberculosis. Meanwhile, Koch and Emmy were having marital problems.

Divorce

In June 1893, Koch and Emmy decided to divorce; and two months later, in a move that shocked many within the German medical community, forty-year-old Koch married eighteen-year-old Hedwig Freiberg, a pretty young German artist.[222] Soon after, Koch was offered the directorship of an Institute for Infectious Diseases (called the Koch Institute today) in Berlin. He accepted and was able to devote all his time to studying infectious diseases.

Rinderpest Disease

In 1896, Koch was contacted by the South African government and asked to study *rinderpest* or "cattle plague" in that country. The symptoms of the disease include chills, difficulty breathing, fever, and death among infected animals. When he arrived in South Africa, Koch found the task difficult because he could neither see the microbes in his microscope nor grow them in a test tube.[223] After three months' work, Koch was able to discover how to stop the disease from spreading from wild animal herds to cattle, but he was not able to discover its cause. Today, scientists know that rinderpest is caused by a virus rather than a bacterium, and it was not possible to see the virus until the electron microscope was invented. Koch found that healthy animals could be made immune by injecting them with a vaccine made from the blood of cattle who had contracted the disease and survived. The primitive vaccine was 75 percent effective in preventing rinderpest and saved millions of cattle in South Africa.[224] He next studied malaria when an outbreak occurred in Rome.

Malaria

Malaria is transmitted when a female anopheles mosquito that has ingested blood from an infected person lands on a healthy person and transmits the parasite while extracting blood. Koch discovered how to tell whether a patient had active or latent malaria by examining a drop of blood under a microscope.[225] He found that if parasites are present in a drop of the patient's blood, malaria is active. Koch also determined the proper dose of quinine for active or latent malarial victims. Malaria can appear seven days after an infection, or it may take a year before symptoms such as chills, fever, convulsions, jaundice, seizure, or mental confusion occur. Koch was internationally recognized for his work on germs and disease when he received the Nobel Prize.

Nobel Prize

Koch was awarded the Nobel Prize in 1905 for his distinguished service to the field of bacteriology.[226] In 1908, he took a trip to England, America, and Japan with his wife Hedwig. In America, he was honored by the German medical society for his work on bacteriology and met his brother for the first time in decades. In June 1908, Koch set sail for Japan where a Shinto temple was built in his honor.

Last Years

By 1907, Koch was beginning to experience mild heart pains when he hiked in the mountains. In March 1910, he had a painful feeling of suffocation in his chest; and a month later, he suffered a near-fatal heart attack after retiring for the night. Koch survived the attack after being treated with morphine, coffee, and compresses on his chest. He traveled to Baden-Baden for a vacation later that year. While on vacation, he quietly died from a heart attack on May 27, 1910.[227] Koch was cremated, his ashes stored in an urn, and the urn was placed in a small niche at the Robert Koch Institute in Berlin.

Chapter 10

————— ✣ —————

X-RAY: WILHELM ROENTGEN

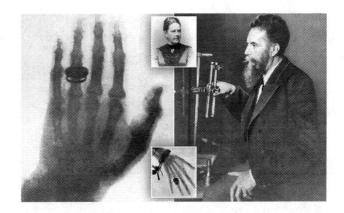

Wilhelm Roentgen wanted to know what would happen when he passed a strong electrical current through a cathode ray tube. To his surprise, he discovered that the rays generated by his more powerful cathode tube caused fluorescence over a meter away while ordinary cathode rays only traveled a few inches. Roentgen also found that when he held a small lead disk with his thumb and finger between the cathode tube and a screen, he could see not only a dark outline of the lead disk but also an image of the bones in his thumb and finger! Roentgen had discovered a ray that could produce an image of the human skeleton on a screen or photographic plate. He called his discovery X-rays, and in 1901, he was awarded the Nobel Prize for his invention. X-rays made treating fractures, bullet wounds, and internal injuries easier and revolutionized the practice of orthopedic surgery.

Roentgen was born on March 27, 1845, in Lennep, Prussia. When he was three, his parents moved to Apeldoorn, Holland, where he attended a primary school and a private boarding school. On December 27, 1862, he enrolled in Utrecht Technical School to prepare for college.[228] Roentgen studied algebra, geometry, physics, chemistry, and technology at Utrecht, but was forced to leave the school when a classmate drew an unflattering picture of their head teacher on the blackboard, and Roentgen was caught looking at the picture when the teacher walked into the room. He refused to disclose who had drawn the picture and was expelled. Roentgen was allowed to audit classes, but he wanted to enroll in a regular university program, so he sent a transcript of his grades in mathematics to the Federal Institute of Technology in Zurich.

The director allowed Roentgen to enroll without taking an entrance examination because his grades in mathematics were so high.[229] He thrived at the Federal Institute of Technology and enjoyed hiking and mountain climbing in his spare time. Roentgen studied mathematics, technical drawing, technology, metallurgy, hydrology, thermodynamics, and mechanical engineering at the Federal Institute. He was a diligent student and earned good grades in engineering and mathematics, passed the written and oral examinations at the institute, and received his diploma on August 6, 1868. Roentgen decided he was not that interested in engineering and went to see a young physics professor named August Kundt to discuss what he should do next. Kundt asked Roentgen what he wanted to do, and he said, "I don't know."

Kundt suggested that Roentgen might find physics interesting, but he said he knew little about the subject. The professor told him he could catch up in physics easily, given his background in mathematics and engineering, and should give the area a try. Roentgen agreed to study physics and work in Kundt's laboratory, exploring the properties of gasses at different temperatures and pressures.[230] His experiments were successful enough that Roentgen was encouraged to submit them as his doctoral dissertation in physics. A physicist and an astronomer examined his dissertation and agreed that Roentgen's work showed adequate knowledge and independent research ability in the field of physics to justify awarding him a graduate degree.

Having earned a degree in engineering and a PhD in physics, Roentgen went to see Anna Bertha Ludwig, the girl he loved, to make plans for their future. However, his parents were not sure they wanted a Swiss girl in the family, so they cautioned Roentgen not to do anything about his marriage plans before they had a chance to know her better. Roentgen reluctantly postponed his marriage and joined Kundt as the first assistant, helping him in the physics laboratory. Working in Kundt's laboratory offered Roentgen the opportunity to learn experimental physics, and the professor was delighted with Roentgen's experimental techniques and careful attention to detail. In 1870, Kundt was offered the chair of physics at the University of Würzburg, which he accepted. He invited Roentgen to join him as his first assistant, but Roentgen was reluctant to leave Zurich and Bertha. They finally decided Roentgen should go to Würzburg with Kundt while Bertha went to live with his parents in Holland so she and his family could get to know each other.[231]

University of Würzburg

The physics laboratory at Wurzburg was primitive, but Roentgen made the best of what was available and began a series of experiments studying specific heat (the quantity of energy required to raise the temperature of one gram of a substance one degree Celsius) at constant pressure and volume. In the course of his work, Roentgen found an error in the calculations made by German physicist Friedrich Kohlrausch but waited because he wanted to confirm the error before publishing his findings. After several months, Roentgen was certain Kohlrausch had made an error, so he wrote his observations in a short article and submitted the paper to Kundt, hoping he would approve it for publication. Kundt accepted the paper and sent Roentgen back to the laboratory to continue his experiments. After waiting months for an answer from Kundt, Roentgen was surprised to discover a copy of the *Annalen der Physik und Chemie* open on the desk to his published paper. Kundt had recommended that Roentgen's paper be published in the official journal of the scientific society, and the editors accepted it.[232] He was proud of the publication and anxious to marry Bertha because they had been separated for months and he was lonely. Roentgen's parents finally agreed to their marriage, so he went to Holland to see Bertha and make arrangements.

Marriage

The wedding took place on January 19, 1872, at Roentgen's family home in Apeldoorn, Holland. The occasion was a major festival in the small Dutch village, and everyone was invited to the reception after the wedding. Local musicians played while the guests ate, drank, and danced until dawn.[233] The couple moved into an apartment near the University of Wurzburg, but needed financial assistance from Roentgen's father to make ends meet until he was promoted. Roentgen worked hard, attended Professor Kundt's lectures, and read widely in the new field of electricity. Professor Kundt accepted a teaching and research position at Kaiser Wilhelm University in Strasbourg, beginning April 1, 1872, and asked Roentgen to join him as his first assistant. Roentgen was unhappy with the laboratory facilities at Wurzburg and agreed to continue working with Professor Kundt in Strasbourg.

University of Strasbourg

Roentgen found the equipment in the new physics laboratory much better than at the prior university and was delighted with the change. In 1873, Roentgen published two papers titled "Determination of the Ratio of the Specific Heats at Constant Pressure to Those for Constant Volume in Some Gasses" and the second "On Soldering of Platinum-plated Glasses." In 1874, Roentgen was appointed lecturer for physics and began teaching students for a fee, so his finances improved dramatically. Roentgen was busy during those years. He constructed simple laboratory devices to demonstrate basic physics principles for his students; lectured on the basic principles and facts of physics; published his own experiments on electricity, crystals, and radiation; and wrote articles with Kundt on optics and acoustics. In April 1875, Roentgen was offered a full professorship in physics and mathematics at the Agricultural Academy in Hohenheim.[234] He was interested in having his own department and earning more money but was reluctant to leave Strasbourg and Kundt. However, after long discussions with Professor Kundt and Bertha, he decided to accept the position in Hohenheim.

Roentgen was disappointed when he arrived at the academy because the laboratory was inferior, the university authorities were reluctant to spend money on research equipment, and he had little time for research because of extensive teaching duties. He wrote Kundt about his situation, and the professor invited Roentgen to return to Strasbourg and continue working with him. Roentgen returned as an associate professor of theoretical physics at Strasburg. Kundt and Roentgen published articles on the existence of electromagnetic rotation in gasses, measured its angle of rotation, and then submitted the work for publication. After several years of working with Kundt in Strasburg, the chair of physics at the University of Giessen became vacant, and several colleagues suggested Roentgen should apply for the post. He visited Giessen, was impressed with the university, and accepted the position of professor and director of physical science at Giessen.

University of Giessen

Located thirty miles north of Frankfurt, Giessen was an ancient university town with inviting hills for hiking and good research facilities when Roentgen joined the staff.[235] He continued studying the effect of heat on crystals but often became so interested in a new idea while he was at Giessen that he would begin a totally different line of experiments and neglect submitting his prior studies for publication. As a result, several of Roentgen's experiments were not published until years after he completed the original work. In 1888, Roentgen proved that a magnetic effect is produced when a dielectric glass plate is passed between two electrically charged condensers. Faraday and Maxwell had predicted the result, based on their theory of electromagnetism, and Roentgen confirmed their theoretical prediction experimentally. This discovery solidified Roentgen's reputation as a first-class experimental physicist, and other physicists began sending him papers for comment. Professor Heinrich Hertz sent Roentgen a paper describing his work on electric oscillation, a phenomenon that would eventually lead Roentgen to discover the X-ray.

University of Würzburg

In 1888, Roentgen was offered the position of full professor of physical science and director of a new physics institute at the University of Würzburg.[236] The physics institute had constructed new classrooms, a lecture hall, a laboratory space, and a private apartment for the director and his family. When Roentgen first visited the physics institute, he was so impressed with the research, teaching, and living facilities that he accepted the position immediately. Over the next six years, he published several important papers in physics and became even more respected. His teaching duties included courses in mechanics, acoustics, and optics. Roentgen developed exercises for the elementary physics laboratory and advised graduate students about their research. He continued studying the effects of pressure on the properties of solids and liquids, exploring the compressibility of liquids such as alcohol and ether, and measuring the dielectric constant (the ratio of the electric permeability of materials under pressure to the permeability of the same material in a vacuum). He also began exploring the properties of cathode rays, which produced his most important invention.

Cathode Rays

The study of electricity began when the English natural scientist William Gilbert published research on magnetism and static electricity at the beginning of the seventeenth century. He showed that magnetic forces produce circular motions associated with the earth's rotation. Gilbert's

early ideas about electricity were extended and clarified by Benjamin
Franklin, Luigi Galvani, Alessandro Volta, Andre Ampere, Greg Ohm,
Michael Faraday, and Joseph Henry over the next two centuries.[237] The
cathode ray tube was developed after Evangelista Torricelli, and Otto von
Guericke invented the vacuum pump. A few years later, in 1855, Heinrich
Geissler used the vacuum pump to evacuate glass tubes, filled the vacuum
tubes with different gasses, and passed high-voltage electrical discharges
through them. Geissler found that electrons flowed from the cathode end
of the vacuum tube when an electrical current was passed through the
tube. Geissler called the flow of electrons he had discovered "cathode rays."
Roentgen acquired one of Geissler's vacuum tubes, passed a higher-voltage
electrical current through the tube, and discovered X-rays.[238]

He became interested in studying vacuum tubes after Philipp Lenard
reported that cathode rays produce luminescent effects and darken
photographic plates when subjected to high-voltage electricity. Roentgen
was intrigued by this result and began a series of experiments using
vacuum tubes to understand their fundamental properties. He equipped
his laboratory with a Ruhmkorff induction coil, a Hittorf-Crookes vacuum
tube, a Lenard tube, and a Raps vacuum pump. Roentgen attached the
vacuum pump to a tube so he could control pressure in the tube while he
applied varying electrical voltages to it. He expected that decreasing the
pressure inside the cathode tube and increasing the voltage of electrical
current passing through the cathode tube would produce stronger cathode
rays. Roentgen wanted to generate stronger and more focused rays by these
procedures and explore their properties.

X-rays

Roentgen covered his experimental vacuum tube with a black cardboard
box to determine whether the rays he was generating would penetrate its
walls. He found the rays he generated with his new cathode tube passed
through the black cardboard and produced a fluorescent effect on a small
screen painted with barium platinocyanide placed close to the cathode end
of the tube. Based on these results, Roentgen believed he had discovered a

new effect of cathode ray tubes and set out to understand how the new ray worked.[239] He hooked the cathode ray tube to the electrodes of a Ruhmkorff magnetic induction coil, closed the windows to check that the black box was emitting no light, and was preparing to set up a small screen painted with barium platinocyanide close to the cathode end of the tube when he noticed a weak light coming from a nearby table.

Roentgen was puzzled by the light and decided to pass a series of electrical discharges through the tube to explore what was happening. On each occasion, he saw the unexplained fluorescence associated with discharges from the Ruhmkorff magnetic induction coil. Roentgen was surprised and curious about the result and decided to study the phenomenon in detail. He was excited by the effect of his new cathode ray vacuum tube because it was generating a totally new effect, and he wanted to understand the process in detail before he announced the discovery. He lit a match and saw that the mysterious light was coming from a small barium platinocyanide screen lying on a table near the cathode ray tube.

He repeated the experiment several times, moving the screen farther away from the cathode ray tube with each test, and was able to produce the same florescent effect at greater and greater distances. Roentgen was now convinced he had created a totally new type of cathode ray with the Hittorf-Crookes vacuum tube he was using because the effect from the new ray happened at much greater distances than anything observed using ordinary cathode rays. Roentgen knew conventional cathode rays travel only a few centimeters in air, but the ray he was generating was creating a photoluminescent reaction over a meter away from the cathode tube.

He worked all weekend to understand the characteristics of his new ray. After each experiment, Roentgen made detailed notes of the apparatus he had used and his observations of the results for later study. Being a careful observer, and working with a totally new effect, he repeated each experiment several times to confirm his results because the new phenomenon he was seeing was so unusual. Roentgen found it hard to believe what he was observing. After he had demonstrated repeatedly that the rays penetrated more than a meter of air and still created fluorescence on a screen, Roentgen decided to see if the new rays would penetrate other substances besides air.

He began by placing a piece of paper, a playing card, and a book between the experimental cathode tube and the screen. Roentgen found that the new rays passed through all these materials although the fluorescence caused by rays passing through the book was weaker than the fluorescence caused by the rays passing through paper or a playing card. He decided to test the new ray using other materials to see what happened.

Roentgen found that a thin sheet of aluminum diffused the rays about the same amount as a book, but a sheet of lead blocked the rays entirely. Roentgen concluded that the type and thickness of material placed between the vacuum tube and the screen affected the ray's transmission and wanted to explore these results in detail using other materials so he could understand the properties of his new ray and how it penetrated different substances.

Photographing Bones

Roentgen concluded that his new ray was a form of radiation because it traveled in a straight line and cast a regular shadow when passing through different materials. He wanted to understand how lead blocked the new ray and began his next experiment by holding a small disk of lead with his thumb and finger between the cathode ray vacuum tube and the screen. To his surprise, not only could he see the dark outline of the lead disk, but he could also see shadows of the bones in his thumb and finger on the screen in front of the new cathode ray tube. Roentgen was shocked to see images of his bones covered with an outline of tissue projected on the screen in his laboratory.[240] He feared if he published these results, the scientific community would think he was a fool, so Roentgen decided to continue his experiments in secret and share his results with other scientists only after he had repeated and confirmed the findings and understood the new ray more completely.

During most of 1895, Roentgen worked on his new ray to prove to himself it was a repeatable phenomenon rather than a random event. Recalling that cathode rays produced an image on photographic material, he decided to see if the new ray produced by the Hittorf-Crookes vacuum tube would create a similar image on a photographic plate. Roentgen placed a disk of platinum on a photographic plate and exposed it to his ray. The developed photographic plate showed a light area in the shape of the platinum disk, which had absorbed some of the rays. He then did the same experiment with several other materials and photographed the results to confirm that what he was seeing with his own eyes also appeared in the photographic images.

"A New Kind of Ray"

After repeating these experiments several times and becoming convinced the new ray was a reliable and significant finding, Roentgen submitted his work in a paper entitled "A New Kind of Ray" to the editor of the Physical-Medical Society. He sent copies of the printed paper to prominent physicists for their comments.[241] Roentgen also enclosed X-ray photographs of his wife's hand and other objects with his paper to demonstrate the wide range of effects achieved with the "X-ray," as he called his discovery. The reactions from readers of his paper were mixed. Some criticized Roentgen for producing a death ray that could be used to kill people. Others congratulated him for a wonderful discovery that could have important medical applications. A few physicists even said his finding was impossible and he must be mistaken. Roentgen was invited to demonstrate his discovery at the Imperial Court in Berlin before Kaiser Wilhelm. He traveled to Berlin by train on a cold Sunday to see Kaiser Wilhelm and demonstrate his new ray.

When he arrived, Roentgen set up his equipment and demonstrated the properties of X-rays to the kaiser and his guests. With his fluorescent screen, Roentgen demonstrated how X-rays penetrate wood, cardboard, and several other substances, but didn't offer to photograph a human hand because he had only one tube and was concerned it might burn out. He did bring several X-ray photographs of hands that created a sensation when they were passed around. Roentgen was awarded the Prussian Order of the Crown, Second Class by Kaiser Wilhelm, and congratulated by the physicists attending the demonstration for his outstanding discovery.

After this initial public demonstration before Kaiser Wilhelm, Roentgen refused to lecture about his discovery despite repeated requests, wanting to spend his time in the laboratory studying the effect of X-rays on different substances.

However, he couldn't avoid giving a lecture that was already scheduled for January 23, 1896, at the Würzburg Physical-Medical Society. A group of prominent physicists and medical professionals attended, and the hall was packed when Roentgen walked to the podium. The crowd gave him a standing ovation before he could even begin his lecture. When the audience settled down, Roentgen began describing his experiments, cautioning his audience that the studies were preliminary and he needed to do further work to fully understand the X-ray. He gave credit to Hertz and Lenard for their earlier work on the cathode ray tube and then described the fluorescence produced by his X-ray on a barium platinocyanide screen. Next, Roentgen described how he discovered that the new vacuum tube he was using generated radiation that penetrated black paper, wood, and a book. Roentgen said he had used photographic plates to record his results to make certain his eyes were not deceiving him and so others could verify his results for themselves. He wanted to be certain the images he was seeing were real and not an illusion.

Roentgen demonstrated the power of X-rays to penetrate paper, wood, tin, and his own hand during the lecture. He showed the audience various X-ray photographs of weights in a box, a compass, a wire wound around a spool of wood, and an X-ray photograph of a hand. The photographs were passed around, inspected, and praised by those attending Roentgen's lecture.[242] To close his lecture, Roentgen asked the famed anatomist Albert von Kolliker if he could take an X-ray photograph of his hand, and the professor agreed. The X-ray photograph was taken, developed, and shown to the audience. They erupted in loud applause. Professor Kolliker said he had never attended a lecture that presented ideas of such importance to medicine and asked Roentgen if it was possible to take X-ray photographs of other parts of the body to diagnose various diseases. Roentgen said that all human tissue except bones seemed to be of equal density and would not show up clearly on an X-ray photograph.

Medical Applications

Physicians and surgeons expressed keen interest in the X-ray as a diagnostic tool for fractures of bones and to test for dental decay. Surgeons also wanted to study the digestive tract and suggested that if a patient drank an opaque substance such as barium, they could take an X-ray photograph of the gut and determine if there was a blockage. Dr. Hermann Gocht, an orthopedic surgeon at Eppendorf Hospital, reported that initially he had been skeptical of the X-ray but, after reading Roentgen's report, wanted the apparatus available at his hospital. However, there was no source for ordering an X-ray machine until C. H. F. Muller, a maker of vacuum tubes and other electrical equipment, agreed to design and manufacture a practical X-ray machine for medical use and offer it for sale to physicians and hospitals. For his achievement, Roentgen was awarded the honorary title of doctor of medicine by several German universities.[243] The public wanted to know about this new X-ray so newspapers began publishing stories about Roentgen's discovery.

The Popular Press

Newspaper editors recognized that Roentgen's X-ray, his astounding photographs, and the fact that his discovery would help in the diagnosis of disease made an interesting story. An article in the *Frankfurter Zeitung* newspaper, published on January 7, 1896, called his discovery "sensational" and "epoch-making." It explained that Roentgen had taken an evacuated Crookes tube, passed an induction current through it, and taken photographs of objects using rays emitted by the tube. The article stated that ordinary human tissue is transparent to the rays, but bones and metals block the rays, leaving an outline of their structure and shape on photographic plates. The article said that physicians and surgeons were interested in using X-rays to diagnose fractures in bones and study internal diseases.

Reprints of Roentgen's original article were quickly translated into English and French for easier access by foreign physicians. Some Christians argued that X-rays proved the existence of the human spirit, and a farmer in Iowa claimed he had turned base metal into gold by subjecting it to X-rays for three hours. Humor magazines published images showing people dressed in elegant clothes positioned as skeletons at a party or looking through an X-ray device that showed what was happening behind a door. Firms in London offered X-ray opera glasses and X-ray-proof garments for sale. Roentgen was distressed by the newspaper stories sensationalizing his discovery. He said newspapers were not a suitable media for reporting his findings because they were distorting and sensationalizing his invention. The papers ignored him and continued their sensational stories because they sold newspapers. Roentgen soon faced claims that others had discovered X-rays before him.

Priority Claims

Roentgen soon learned that other scientists were claiming they had discovered X-rays before him. Because so little was known about the physical characteristics of X-rays at that time, the prior claims generally involved other electrical phenomena mistakenly attributed to X-rays. Other scientists might well have produced X-rays from Crookes tubes before Roentgen reported his detailed findings in a scientific article, but these earlier scientists had not recognized the importance of this new type of radiation, observed it carefully, and understood its properties. In spite of claims by several scientists that they had discovered or observed X-rays before Roentgen, there is no doubt within the German physics community that Roentgen had made the original discovery that rays from a Crookes tube could penetrate human tissue and produce an image of human bones on photographic plates. The discovery was his alone as far as fellow German physicists were concerned.

For years after Roentgen discovered X-rays, it was difficult to differentiate cathode rays from X-rays, producing confusion and honest disputes among scientists. Some claimed that X-rays and cathode rays were both electromagnetic phenomena, but Roentgen disagreed. He believed X-rays had no electrical charge, so cathode rays and X-rays must be fundamentally different. Roentgen admitted he didn't know what X-rays actually were, but said he was trying to understand them by continuing his experiments. He speculated that X-rays were longitudinal waves similar to sound waves but of higher frequency because he was unable to refract X-rays with the materials available at the time. It was not until 1912 that Max von Laue was able to show X-rays are a form of electromagnetic radiation similar to light by using crystals to refract X-rays and produce diffraction. Von Laue won the Nobel Prize for his work in 1914.[244] Meanwhile, physicians and surgeons were discovering new uses for X-rays almost daily.

Medical Diagnoses

X-ray photographs attracted public attention because they showed images no one had seen before. Many early X-ray photographs were of the hand, but Roentgen soon produced a photograph of a broken forearm, which he sent to the editor of the *British Medical Journal* on February 15, 1896, to show the value of X-rays in the diagnosis of fractures. Dr. Franz Koenig took an X-ray photograph of his assistant's hand, showing a piece of glass from an exploding tank that had become embedded in his skin. Other X-ray photographs showed a needle embedded in a girl's hand and a deformed bone in the right hand of a boy. X-ray pictures of teeth were taken by placing film, wrapped to protect it from light, in the person's mouth and exposing it to X-rays. F. Kurlbaum and W. Wien made X-ray photographs showing large nodes and damaged joints in the hands of arthritis patients. Other physicians began having patients drink solutions of opaque liquids such as barium so they could take X-ray photographs of the stomach and intestines to diagnose blockages. Dr. E. Neusser photographed kidney stones, bladder stones, and gallstones using X-rays. The medical uses of X-rays seemed almost unlimited.

The first private X-ray laboratory in the world opened in London on March 11, 1896, and the New York Post-Graduate Medical School and Hospital and the Hahnemann Hospital in Chicago established X-ray departments at their institutions the same year. In January 1897, the Belgian government recommended that all hospitals in the country establish X-ray departments equipped to take photographs for use in diagnosing medical disorders. X-ray photographs of famous people created sensations when they were published showing abnormalities. Engineers believed X-rays could be used to test for flaws in metals, and governments rushed to test their war equipment for flaws.

Metal Imperfections

One of the early photographs Roentgen took was of his shotgun, and he suggested X-rays could be used to examine metal objects to determine if they contained flaws that might cause a failure. The German and Austrian war ministries recognized the importance of using X-rays to examine guns and armor plating for defects before employing them in combat.[245] Arthur Wright of Yale University x-rayed a piece of welded steel and suggested the method could be used to determine if the welds were sound. The Carnegie Steel Works began using X-rays to test steel the company produced in 1896. Thomas Edison discovered that X-rays could increase the hardness of certain metals. Post office authorities in France used X-rays to detect explosives sent through the mail. Geologists speculated that X-rays might help them detect deposits of coal and iron ore underground. Jewelers used X-rays to distinguish real gems from fakes. There seemed no end to the use of X-rays, especially as the equipment improved and became more powerful.

Demand for X-ray tubes increased quickly, and companies developed improved vacuum tubes for use in medical diagnosis and metal testing. Because of rapid improvements in X-ray technology, rays capable of penetrating a foot of steel were soon available. Book publishers offered collections of X-ray photographs of human skeletons, a human liver, a stomach, a heart, a finger, a broken arm, a foot crushed by a horse, and a white fish with visible fins. Roentgen refused to patent his invention, saying X-rays should be freely available to the public although the decision cost him a fortune. Thomas Edison encouraged others to study Roentgen's invention and see if they could profit by developing and patenting new methods of producing X-rays or new procedures for using the device. X-rays were so popular it soon became clear that continued exposure could harm human tissue.

Dangers of X-rays

While working with X-rays, Roentgen placed a lead shield between himself and the X-ray tube to make the images he photographed sharper and avoid fogging spare photographic plates in his laboratory. Because of these precautions, Roentgen avoided suffering any harmful effects of X-rays, but not all early users were so careful. The cautious ones believed that because X-rays were powerful, they might have harmful effects on the human body and thought it prudent to protect themselves with a lead shield. After X-rays were in use for a few months, L. G. Stevens in England reported that prolonged exposure to X-rays produced damage to the skin similar to a sunburn.[246] Other scientists reported that when the skull was X-rayed, patients often lost hair at the spot where the X-rays were concentrated.

H. D. Hawks gave public demonstrations of X-rays at Bloomingdale's Department Store in New York for two or three hours every day, showing the bones of his hand to shoppers. In a few weeks, Hawks noticed dryness of the skin on his hand, and he developed what appeared to be a bad sunburn on the hand that had been exposed to X-rays. A week later, his fingernails stopped growing. Hawks sought medical attention to relieve the pain from his burns and tried wearing gloves to protect his hand, but they didn't help. Injuries happened because there was no pain or other sensation indicating that the X-rays were harming human tissue. X-rays can't be seen, smelled, tasted, felt, or heard and there was no pain while the burn was occurring, so demonstrators and physicians exposed themselves to dangerous levels of radiation without realizing they were being harmed.[247]

X-rays attracted the attention of military physicians treating wounded soldiers because they could determine the exact location of a bullet and the extent of injury to bones quickly and easily using the device. A report by the American Army Medical Corps during the Spanish-American War noted that the use of X-rays on bullet wounds was invaluable because the location of a bullet could be determined precisely and removed easily.

Only two instances of radiation burns were reported during the Spanish-American War in Cuba, possibly from prolonged exposure or a defective tube. Surgeons began to realize that the length of exposure, the nearness of the X-ray tube to the skin, and the health of a patient all contributed to the intensity of radiation burns from prolonged or repeated exposure to X-rays.

An attorney used X-ray evidence in a personal injury case of a dancer who fell and injured her foot between performances. The attorney took X-ray photographs of both her feet and the difference in the bone structure of the two feet convinced a judge she had indeed been injured. Medical experts who testified in personal injury cases before a court immediately recognized how valuable an X-ray photograph could be in their work and began using them extensively when testifying.

Roentgen published a final summary of his research on March 10, 1897, in a Prussian Academy of Sciences journal, entitled "Further Observations on the Properties of X-rays—Third Communication." The early part of this final paper described the properties of X-rays, listed the transparencies of various materials to X-rays, and compared these penetrations to a standard aluminum plate. The middle section of his article described experiments with soft and hard X-rays (those generated with low energy were called soft X-rays and those generated with high energy were called hard X-rays). Hard X-rays can be used to create images of more opaque objects because they penetrate thicker or more dense materials. Roentgen was about to receive the ultimate scientific prize for his work on X-rays.

Nobel Prize

After he published his "Third Communication," Roentgen returned to teaching and discussing X-rays with his students and colleagues, but stopped studying the new ray himself. He continued to accumulate prizes, and several scientific societies made him an honorary member. The Bavarian government offered him the title of "von," which he refused, and the city of Munich offered him the post as head of the physical science institute at the University of Munich, which he accepted. His duties as head of the institute included lecturing on experimental physics and guiding graduate students' research. Roentgen was awarded the Nobel Prize for physics in 1901 based on his discovery of X-rays.[248] He traveled to Stockholm to accept the prize and willed the forty-one thousand dollars he received to the University of Würzburg for scientific research. Bertha developed a cough, and her health began slowly declining a few years after Roentgen received the Nobel Prize.

Health Issues

By 1919, Bertha's health had deteriorated to the point where she could hardly leave her bed. She was suffering from heart and kidney insufficiency, and the medications she took did little except make her comfortable. She died on October 31, 1919. Roentgen was devastated by her death and began preparing for his own end soon after. He organized his papers for later publication and distributed materials associated with his discovery of the X-ray to various museums. Roentgen donated the original Hittorf-Crookes vacuum tube used in his first experiments with X-rays to the German museum in Munich and left instructions for his ashes to be buried alongside his wife Bertha in the cemetery at Giessen. In late 1922 and early 1923, Roentgen began to suffer gastrointestinal pains. He was certain he had developed intestinal cancer, but a physician told him there was no cancer and he didn't know what was wrong.

Roentgen continued to lose weight and was unable to concentrate or see well enough to continue his research. On February 7, 1923, Roentgen was feeling ill so he contacted his physician and asked him to come for a consultation, but the doctor was too busy. He suggested Roentgen take opium and he would see him later that evening. When the doctor arrived, Roentgen looked terrible so the physician gave him a sedative and put the man to bed. The next day, Roentgen felt better and insisted he wanted to get up. He tried to sit in his favorite chair to read the newspaper but was too weak. That afternoon, Roentgen vomited, and his physician diagnosed a blocked intestine. Roentgen died on February 10, 1923, in his bed.[249] The entire world mourned the loss of Germany's great scientist and discoverer of the X-ray.

Chapter 11

INSULIN: FREDERICK BANTING

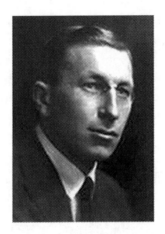

F rederick Banting decided to include a discussion of diabetes in a lecture to university students. While preparing the lecture, he began to wonder if secretions from the pancreas might be responsible for controlling blood sugar levels. Banting decided to isolate the secretion produced by the islets of Langerhans and see if it would help manage diabetes. After months of work, Banting and Charles Best were able to produce an extract from the islet of Langerhans that regulated blood sugar in diabetic dogs. However, they needed a way to produce large quantities of what came to be called "insulin." Banting tested the safety of insulin by injecting it under his own skin and suffered no adverse effects. He also found a way to produce large quantities of insulin from mature beef pancreas tissue and contracted with Eli Lilly, a US pharmaceutical company, to manufacture the drug. Clinical trials of insulin produced by Lilly were successful, and the drug was approved for the treatment of diabetes by the US Food and Drug Administration. In 1923, Banting was awarded the Nobel Prize for his discovery. Insulin has allowed millions of diabetic people to live normal lives.

Banting was born on November 15, 1891, in Alliston, Canada. In the summer, he worked on his father's farm, fished, and hunted; in the winter, he skated on the Boyne River. Banting didn't like school because he was shy and had trouble speaking in class. He entered the University of Toronto at nineteen and then attended the University of Toronto Medical School.[250] Banting studied hard in medical school but earned only average grades. When England declared war on Germany in 1914, he enlisted in the Canadian Army Medical Service and was sent to Europe to treat wounded soldiers. Early in the war, Banting was stationed at a seaside hospital to treat victims of poison gas. Later, he was transferred to France as part of a medical team assigned to an ambulance at the front, cleaning and bandaging wounds to stop bleeding and prevent shock before sending injured soldiers to a field hospital or home to England.[251] He was subjected to cannon fire while tending the wounded, but it didn't seem to bother him.

One day, he and another doctor were smoking at the entrance to a dugout when they saw a dog running across the battlefield. They were concerned the dog might be carrying a German Army message and set out to capture it. When they caught the dog, they saw it was only a stray; so they fed it, gave the animal water, and it adopted them. Later, as they were standing in front of their bunker, the dog howled, and the two doctors ducked into their dugout just before a German shell landed where they had been standing. The dog's keen hearing had saved their lives.

After the war, Banting was posted to Christie Street Hospital in Toronto to treat wounded soldiers suffering from damaged or diseased bones. Later, he worked as a senior surgeon at the Hospital for Sick Children in Toronto before establishing his own private medical practice. After practicing medicine for a while, Banting became interested in research, so he looked around for an opportunity to work in a laboratory. To earn extra money, he lectured at Western University in London, Ontario. While preparing a lecture on carbohydrate metabolism, he decided to include a discussion of diabetes to make his presentation more interesting.

Banting knew food was digested by enzymes produced in the pancreas and that another secretion produced by the islets of Langerhans went directly into the bloodstream, but no one was certain what the second secretion did. In the nineteenth century, German surgeons had discovered that if a dog's pancreas was removed, it became diabetic, so Banting wondered if one of the pancreatic enzymes might be associated with regulating blood sugar. He decided to learn how pancreatic enzymes worked and in the process discovered an effective treatment for diabetes.

Research on Diabetes

Banting knew diabetic patients were constantly hungry and thirsty, had little energy, eventually fell into a coma, and died because doctors could do little to manage their erratic blood sugar levels. Patients with diabetes accumulated too much sugar in their blood because it was not absorbed into their cells for some unknown reason. Because there was excess sugar in the diabetic's blood, it spilled over into the kidneys, triggering them to produce extra urine to excrete the sugar. Because the kidneys were producing so much urine, the patient was always thirsty; and because the diabetic patient's body was not absorbing sugar, he or she always felt hungry. Living with diabetes was a constant struggle to stay alive; diabetic patients' skin became dry, their hair was brittle, and they often became blind or developed infections in their legs or feet that required treatment or amputation. Special low-calorie diets were prescribed to manage diabetes, but nothing seemed to help.

During his preparation of the lecture on carbohydrate metabolism, Banting read an article in the journal *Surgery, Gynecology, and Obstetrics* concerning the function of the islets of Langerhans and diabetes. He knew the islets of Langerhans were small clusters of cells found in the pancreas, and some physicians had suggested they might produce an enzyme that could control blood sugar.[252] Banting was fascinated by the article and decided to extract this unknown secretion from the islets of Langerhans and see if it could be used to treat diabetes. He planned to tie off the duct that connected a dog's pancreas to its stomach and keep the dog alive until all the pancreatic cells degenerated, leaving behind the living islets of Langerhans. Banting would then extract the islets of Langerhans from the animal, isolate the secretion produced by the islets, and determine if the unknown secretion could be used to treat diabetes.

He decided the idea was worth pursuing, so Banting contacted an expert on diabetes at the University of Toronto named J. J. R. Macleod. He scheduled an appointment with Macleod and told him about his idea. Macleod was skeptical but decided to let Banting explore the idea in his laboratory because even if it didn't work, the failure would eliminate another theory about what caused diabetes. Also, there was a chance Banting's idea might yield interesting results. Macleod told him to come back in six months, and he would help Banting establish a laboratory at the University of Toronto to do research on diabetes.

Working with Macleod

Banting wondered if Macleod would remember the promise to him in six months, but when he called, the professor honored his agreement and helped Banting set up a laboratory. Macleod gave Banting space on the top floor of his research laboratory and assigned him a bright medical student named Charles Best to help with the research.[253] Banting and his assistant cleaned the space and set to work. At first, they had trouble keeping the dogs alive because the animals often bled to death or died quickly from infections until they learned how to operate properly. The work was tedious because each dog had to be anesthetized, cut open, the pancreatic duct tied off, the incision closed, and then they had to wait for the animal to recover and the pancreas to degenerate before they could remove the islets of Langerhans and extract the mysterious secretion to test on diabetic dogs.

Banting believed it was essential for the pancreas to degenerate because otherwise, he thought its powerful enzyme might contaminate or destroy the substances secreted by the islet of Langerhans. Every few weeks,

Banting would remove a degenerated pancreas containing the living islets of Langerhans, chop it up, and place the tissue in a mortar containing ice-cold Ringer's solution (a mixture of water and salts used to preserve tissue). He then ground the islets tissue and Ringer's solution in a mortar, filtered it through cheesecloth to collect the liquid from the islet of Langerhans, and injected the liquid into a diabetic dog with no pancreas. Banting wanted to determine whether the extract from the islet of Langerhans would control the blood sugar levels in a diabetic dog. If the extract from the islets of Langerhans controlled blood sugar levels in a diabetic dog, he planned to try the extract on humans to see if it would cure diabetes.

Banting found it difficult to ligate the small pancreatic ducts in dogs; sometimes the incision didn't heal, or the dogs didn't become diabetic following surgery because the pancreas hadn't fully degenerated. Even more frustrating, the liquid extract they produced from the islet of Langerhans didn't control the blood sugar levels in dogs with no pancreas. Banting and Best were getting discouraged but continued trying to develop a treatment for diabetes. Finally, in August 1921, they produced an extract from the islet of Langerhans that controlled the blood sugar level in a dog with no pancreas. They repeated the procedure several times to confirm that the extract did indeed control blood sugar levels in dogs without a pancreas.[254]

They were still a long way from finding a workable treatment for diabetes because making the extract was so slow it was impossible to produce enough extract to treat thousands of human diabetics. Banting and Best had made progress because the extract from the islet of Langerhans did control blood sugar levels in dogs with no pancreas, and the dogs showed no signs of diabetes while they were receiving the liquid extract. Moreover, when they stopped injecting the liquid extract from the islets of Langerhans into diabetic dogs with no pancreas, they died. It appeared the substance from the islets of Langerhans did manage blood sugar levels. But how could they make the substance in large enough quantities to treat hundreds of human diabetics?

When Macleod returned to Toronto from his vacation, Banting told him about their results with the extract that seemed to treat diabetes in dogs. Macleod was cautious but interested and asked Banting several probing questions, such as could it be something else lowering the dog's blood sugar, or had he left a small piece of the pancreas in the dog that was keeping it alive? Satisfied with Banting's answers, Macleod told him to continue the research, but Banting complained that the lab was a mess and he was tired of not being paid. Best privately advised Banting to calm down and not anger Macleod because he was the director of the laboratory, and without him, they could not continue their work. To Best's surprise, Macleod agreed to improve the laboratory and hire a part-time assistant to clean it. Banting and Best were also given salaries, and Banting was hired as an assistant in the pharmacology department to earn additional income. With this new arrangement, Banting and Best set about trying to find a more efficient way to produce more of the liquid extract from the islets of Langerhans.

Fetal Animals

Banting began considering other ways to make the liquid extract from the islet of Langerhans in larger quantities. He recalled that farmers often bred their cattle before selling them for slaughter because the animals gained more weight if they were pregnant. He also remembered that the islets of Langerhans developed early in fetal animals and might produce secretions that regulated blood sugar in the fetus before the pancreas began to function. Banting reasoned that without a functioning pancreas, there would be no strong digestive enzymes to destroy the extract from the islet of Langerhans, so he decided to try producing the liquid extract from fetal pancreatic tissue because that would allow him to avoid the complex operation and lengthy wait required before he could produce the liquid extract from mature dogs' islets of Langerhans. Best and Banting bought nine fetal calves from a slaughterhouse and set to work extracting the immature pancreas from them. They produced a liquid extract from the fetal pancreases and tested it to see if it would control blood sugar in dogs without a pancreas. They were able to produce enough extract to treat several diabetic dogs and found that the extract from the fetal calves did control diabetes in dogs with no pancreas.[255] Word of Banting's research spread, and Dr. Elliot Joslin, a prominent physician who treated diabetic patients, contracted Macleod to learn about Banting's research. He was impressed with the results.

Banting injected the liquid extract under his own skin and suffered no adverse reaction, so he concluded it was safe to use the liquid extract on diabetic humans. Macleod suggested they mix the extract with alcohol, evaporate the mixture, and then dissolve it in a salt solution to produce a pure injectable extract to test on human subjects. While Best was purifying the extract, Banting continued to look for a better method to produce larger quantities of the liquid extract. He decided to try making the extract from mature beef pancreases because he could make more that way and treat several dogs at once. Using mature beef pancreases worked, and Banting believed he had found a ready source of the extract to control blood sugar levels in diabetic human patients. Macleod suggested they name the extracted substance *insulin*, and they agreed. Banting wanted to have a chemist on the team who could help them purify insulin and make the procedure more efficient.

Collip Joins the Team

Banting asked Macleod to invite J. B. Collip, a biochemist with experience separating substances from animal tissue, to help them discover a more efficient manufacturing procedure for producing insulin. Macleod contacted Collip, and he agreed to join the research team and try to develop an effective and reliable procedure for extracting insulin from beef pancreatic tissue.[256] On December 22, 1921, Collip tested the pancreatic extract he had developed to see if it would control diabetes in a human patient, but the extract was too weak. They had to make a more concentrated form of insulin. Macleod decided they needed to announce their discovery to claim priority for the invention, so he scheduled a presentation of Banting and Best's work at Yale University.

Announcing the Discovery

On December 30, 1921, Banting presented their results at the American Physiological Society conference at Yale University in New Haven, Connecticut. His paper was titled "The Beneficial Influences of Certain Pancreatic Extracts on Pancreatic Diabetes." Many important doctors who worked on diabetes attended his presentation. Banting was so anxious he had a difficult time presenting his research, and Macleod had to answer questions and help him defend the research after the talk finished. Banting was upset because he had done most of the work on discovering a treatment for diabetes but felt that Macleod was being given the major credit because he was the laboratory director and better known. Banting's sensitivity would create serious problems for him over the years.

On January 11, 1922, Banting and Best went to Toronto General Hospital to supervise the injection of insulin in a fourteen-year-old charity patient with diabetes. The boy's blood sugar level dropped for a while, but the extract produced no beneficial clinical effects. Moreover, the boy developed an abscess at the site of the injection, so they needed to purify the extract before using it on human patients. Macleod suggested Banting purify the insulin by mixing the beef pancreas tissue with alcohol at different concentrations to separate the active insulin from inactive impurities.

Purifying the Extract

On January 16, 1922, Collip succeeded in purifying the liquid extract following Macleod's suggestion. He produced a nearly pure sample of the insulin by gradually increasing the concentration of alcohol. Collip found that the active insulin stayed in solution at higher and higher concentrations of alcohol while the impurities precipitated out of the alcohol and were easy to extract using a centrifuge. On January 23, the diabetic boy in Toronto General Hospital, who had slipped into a coma, was injected with five cubic centimeters of the purified extract, and he quickly revived.[257] Banting, Best, Collip, and Macleod were finally able to manufacture a pure, safe, and effective treatment for human diabetes!

A few days later, Banting saw Collip in the hall at their laboratory and asked how he had purified the extract. Collip told him he wouldn't share the information but said he had told Macleod, and the secret was safe with them. Collip said Macleod had told him he didn't have to disclose his procedure to Banting and Best. Banting also thought he heard Collip say he intended to patent the method himself. Banting flew into a rage and struck Collip in the face with his fist. Best pulled Banting off Collip, and Macleod made them sign an agreement to stop fighting. Banting and Collip reluctantly agreed to work together under Macleod's supervision to perfect the pancreatic extract, and they promised not to patent the method individually.

Macleod presented the team's new results at a conference of the Association of American Physicians in Washington, DC, on May 3, 1922. He summarized their methods, described the results, and used the name "insulin" for the first time in public. Macleod claimed that insulin controls the metabolism of diabetic animals, including humans, and was an effective treatment for human diabetes. He cautioned that producing insulin on a large scale to treat hundreds of diabetic patients was still a challenge, but they hoped to make a breakthrough in the next few months and have insulin available in sufficient quantities to treat hundreds of diabetic patients. The audience stood at the end of Macleod's presentation in honor of their discovery. Banting, Best, Collip, and Macleod were listed as authors of the paper in alphabetical order, but Banting felt slighted because the original idea was his alone and he resented Collip and Macleod sharing credit for his discovery.

Demand for insulin grew quickly as desperate diabetic patients traveled from all over North America seeking treatment. Many of these patients had only weeks to live, but the team was having production problems: Collip had not written down the steps in his procedure and could not remember how to repeat the process. He tried to produce additional insulin, but for some reason, it was weak and didn't control blood sugar levels in diabetic humans. They were unable to produce full-strength insulin, and patients were dying on a daily basis. Banting was furious with Collip, concerned about the diabetic deaths, and began drinking heavily to control his anger and depression.

Banting told Best he wanted to go to the United States because he felt betrayed by Macleod and Collip. Best said he would go with Banting if that was what he wanted because they were in this together. Reassured by Best's faith in him, Banting stopped drinking, and they set about to rediscover the formula for making effective insulin from beef pancreases. Within two months, Banting and Best were able to produce full-strength insulin in large quantities so they could again treat diabetic patients. Banting sent insulin to Dr. John Williams in Rochester, New York, who was trying to save the life of John Havens, the twenty-two-year-old son of an executive at Eastman Kodak. The insulin Williams received from Banting didn't seem to work; so Banting visited Rochester, suggested he increase the dosage, and the patient's diabetic symptoms disappeared. Banting and Best allocated one-third of the insulin they produced to Toronto General Hospital and two-thirds to Banting for use in his private clinic. However, they needed a larger supply of insulin and decided to contact an American pharmaceutical manufacturing company for help.

Contract with Eli Lilly

Banting, Macleod, Best, and Collip patented their discovery and sold the rights to the University of Toronto for one dollar! They also signed a contract with Eli Lilly and Company, a respected US pharmaceutical manufacturer, to produce insulin in Indianapolis, Indiana.[258] Their agreement limited sales of insulin made by Eli Lilly to the United States and gave Banting, Best, Collip, Macleod, and the University of Toronto exclusive rights to produce and sell insulin to the rest of the world. In June 1922, Banting and Best traveled to Indianapolis to show the chemists at Eli Lilly how to produce insulin. They also supervised the production of the first batch of insulin manufactured by Lilly. In August 1922, clinical trials of Lilly insulin began in the United States, supervised by Dr. Elliott Joslin of Boston, Massachusetts, and Dr. Frederick Allen of Morristown, New Jersey. Approximately fifty men and women suffering from late-stage diabetes were recruited and told they would receive an injection of an experimental drug to treat their illness. Dr. Allen injected insulin into six of the most critical patients first. Their symptoms disappeared, and they felt normal for the first time in years. The clinical trials were successful, and insulin was approved for the treatment of diabetes in the US.

The Diabetic Clinic at Toronto General Hospital, with Banting as attending physician, opened on August 21, 1922, using the insulin produced by Eli Lilly in the United States. A Canadian facility established to produce insulin was not yet operating, and Banting wanted to offer insulin to his Canadian patients as soon as possible. The discovery of insulin changed Banting's life: he received awards, money, and gratitude from grateful patients. One such patient was Elizabeth Hughes, daughter of US secretary of state Charles Evans Hughes. When she came to Banting's clinic in 1922, Elizabeth was emaciated and undersized from following the Allen "starvation" diet. She responded to Banting's insulin treatment immediately and began to thrive.

Banting placed her on a normal diet. She gained weight and grew taller. Drs. Elliot Joslin and Frederick Allen didn't recognize Elizabeth when they came to Toronto to see her. When they had been treating Elizabeth, she was emaciated, depressed, and waiting to die. Now, she was healthy and thriving; it seemed like a miracle. By the fall of 1922, insulin was being administered to diabetic patients all over America and Canada. Whenever Banting spoke at a luncheon of dignitaries or before a group of medical students, he was given a standing ovation. He was appointed professor of medical research at the University of Toronto, and the Canadian House of Commons voted him a lifetime annual annuity of $7,500, enough for Banting to live comfortably and devote himself to research for the rest of his life. He was also nominated for the most sought-after prize in medicine.

Nobel Prize

Banting had returned to his new research laboratory in Toronto after traveling to Europe to meet the king of England when his phone rang. He picked up the receiver, and a friend congratulated Banting for winning the

Nobel Prize.[259] Thinking his friend was joking, Banting hung up. He then glanced at the newspaper on his desk and saw that he and Macleod had indeed been awarded the Nobel Prize. Banting was furious that Macleod was sharing his prize while Best was excluded. Banting announced he was going to refuse the prize because his friend and assistant were not included in the award. Banting's friends became concerned about his attitude, and they asked him to speak with Colonel Albert Gooderham, a member of the university's board. Gooderham told Banting to calm down and think straight. He reminded Banting that no Canadian had ever won a Nobel Prize. (Macleod was a native of Scotland and didn't count.) He told Banting to consider his country and how proud Canadians would be of his accomplishment. Banting listened, changed his mind, decided to accept the prize, and share the money with Best.

Banting sent a telegram to Boston, where Best was giving a lecture to Harvard medical students about insulin, telling him he deserved an equal share of the award money from the Nobel Prize for helping discover insulin. A few days later, Macleod announced he would share his prize money with Collip. On the surface, the bad feelings between Macleod and Banting seemed over, but Banting would resent the fame Macleod garnered by being associated with the discovery of insulin for the rest of his life. Banting began attracting attention from female nurses and socialites as a result of his fame and fortune. One of them interested Banting, and he began dating her.

Marion Robertson

In 1924, Banting began dating the socialite Marion Robertson, and they agreed to marry. However, their wedding plans might have fallen through after Marion received a letter accusing Banting of being a cad. The letter was from a woman Banting had been dating who believed he was going to marry her. When Banting changed his mind, she became furious and sent the hateful letter to Marion. However, the spiteful letter had no effect—they were married on June 4, 1924, at her uncle's home.[260] Frederick and Marion Banting traveled to America for a short vacation where he received an honorary degree from Yale University. In July, they took a trip to the Caribbean as guests of the United Fruit Company, spending two months in Cuba, Jamaica, and Central America before returning to Canada.

At a medical conference he was attending when they returned to Canada, Banting realized he had little in common with Marion; she liked to socialize and dance while he preferred to read detective novels and smoke his pipe in the evenings after working in his laboratory all day. Banting found himself alone in a corner many evenings while Marion danced with other men, which made him jealous. They began to argue constantly. The Bantings returned to Toronto in the fall and moved into a three-story brick-and-sandstone house they built at 46 Bedford Road, just north of the University of Toronto. In 1925, Banting and his wife sailed to Europe to collect his Nobel Prize. Banting thanked the Nobel Committee for awarding the prize to him and Macleod but secretly felt betrayed by his old mentor. After winning the Nobel Prize, Banting wondered what kind of research he wanted to pursue and what to do about his difficult marriage.

Marion was unhappy because Banting often came home smelling of dogs and was not polite to her dinner guests. She wanted to socialize every evening while Banting insisted on staying home, having a quiet dinner, and reading a detective story. He didn't like her friends, believing they were shallow and uninteresting. Banting was also discouraged by the progress of his research. He was trying to find a vaccine for cancer and was having no success. Banting planned to give cancer to chickens and find a vaccine that would protect them, but the project was failing. Physicians now know cancer is several different diseases, and only a few are caused by viruses that can be treated with a vaccine. Banting was not studying those types of cancers, so his research was failing. Banting and his wife were fighting most of the time, and he felt miserable. He wondered what to do about his marriage and how to find a better research idea.

Divorce

Banting and Marion tried to maintain a peaceful facade with friends and family, but things were not going well in their relationship. In Canada during the 1920s, it was nearly impossible to end a bad marriage because of social attitudes and strict laws governing divorce. Proving adultery was the only legal means of obtaining a divorce, and even that was difficult. Respectable people in Canada just didn't divorce no matter how bad their marriage was. Banting began drinking and developed a desire to be a detective writer like Arthur Conan Doyle, creator of Sherlock Holmes. He wrote a detective novel featuring a half-Indian with an interest in chemistry and the logical abilities of Holmes. Publishers rejected the book because the plot was too much like a Sherlock Holmes novel. Banting also began writing his autobiography but never finished the book.

They tried to repair their relationship by having a son, but the baby didn't help. Banting finally told Marion he was unhappy with their marriage and began seeing a writer in Toronto named Blodwen Davies. Banting also hired a private detective to collect evidence of Marion's adulterous activities so he could get a divorce. Banting worried that a divorce might ruin his medical reputation and Marion's social standing in Toronto, but he was desperate to end their toxic relationship and didn't care. Their lawyers finally negotiated a divorce settlement that included a clause designed to keep the agreement private. Banting gave Marion two hundred fifty dollars a month as alimony, custody of their son, and possession of their house. However, the *Toronto Telegram* published a front-page account of the divorce settlement, and Marion's father sued Banting, alleging he was the one having an affair and the evidence collected by Banting's private detectives was false. In spite of the suit, the Banting divorce went through as agreed, but a serious financial crisis was just around the corner.

Great Depression

In late 1929, the New York Stock Exchange collapsed, banks shut their doors, investors and depositors lost their money, factories closed, and millions of Americans were thrown out of work. Farmers could not sell their crops or pay their mortgages, and banks foreclosed on thousands of farms. The Great Depression spread around the world. Banting believed the Great Depression was proof that capitalism didn't work, and he thought the

Soviet Union had found a better way to organize the world economy. He also liked how the Soviet Union controlled the press so it could not criticize authorities or pry into personal matters. Banting traveled to Europe in 1933 to attend the International Cancer Congress in Madrid, Spain, in connection with his research.

Banting continued to receive honors and awards for his work on insulin and his career and was unaffected by the divorce. In June 1934, he was awarded the title of Knight Commander of the Civil Order of the British Empire for his discovery of insulin. Although the title made him uncomfortable, it proved he was not disgraced and was a welcome affirmation of his continuing professional status. Banting hoped to make another scientific discovery as important as insulin but was unable to develop a good research idea. He believed that coming up with a good idea was like fishing; you had to wait for a fish to strike the lure, but the waiting was worth it if you caught a big fish.

In 1935, Banting was inducted into the Royal Society and traveled to the Soviet Union to attend the Fifteenth Physiological Congress in Leningrad. He was impressed that the Soviet Union had no unemployment in the 1930s while the rest of the world was mired in depression. Many capitalist countries suffered unemployment rates of over 20 percent. Banting met the famous Russian physiologist Ivan Pavlov, who had won a Nobel Prize for his work on the physiology of digestion, and toured his Institute of Experimental Medicine. Pavlov was getting old and complained of poor health. Banting spent most of July 1935 traveling around the Soviet Union, being shown newly built houses and factories by government guides. However, he could not help noticing the shoddy huts of the peasants and the tattered clothes they wore. He also noticed that railway stations had special waiting rooms for foreign travelers and important government officials despite the fact that there were supposed to be no class differences in the Soviet Union. Banting was puzzled by the discrepancies between the Soviet Union's claims and the reality he was seeing with his own eyes but ignored the hypocrisy because he was enamored by the idea of communism and government control of the economy. On his way home, Banting traveled through Europe and was struck by the extensive war preparations in Germany.

Preparing for War

Banting traveled by train through Eastern Europe, saw Nazi flags flying all over Germany, and became alarmed by the possibility of another world war. When he returned to Canada, Banting started studying the use of disease as a war weapon because he was worried about Hitler's buildup of German military forces and believed bacterial warfare might be an effective way to counter the Nazi war machine.[261] He was appointed to Canada's National Research Council, a government bureau established to oversee scientific research related to war preparations. The head of the National Research Council asked Banting to draft a memorandum on biological warfare for discussion at their next meeting. He concluded in his report that it would be feasible to drop a waterborne disease such as cholera into reservoirs from airplanes and that animal-borne diseases could be spread among enemy military and civilian populations by releasing infected animals into the country. The National Research Council reached no conclusion concerning his report, however. Banting toured Canada to study what researchers were doing to prepare for war and pleaded with the Canadian government for more money to support basic medical research. He was busy with government affairs and found little time to work in his laboratory. Banting was depressed about the coming war in Europe, drinking heavily, and his research was going nowhere. A bright spot in his life was a romance with Henrietta Ball.

Banting fell in love with and married Henrietta Ball, a native of Quebec after she came to the University of Toronto to work in the Department of Medical Research. She was twenty-five, and Banting was forty-six when they met. Soon after they married, Hitler invaded Poland, and Banting enlisted as a pathologist in the Canadian Medical Corps. He was promoted to major and ordered to resume his work for the National Research Council even though he volunteered to treat wounded soldiers at the front as he had done during World War I. Banting was concerned that the Germans would infect Allied civilian populations and military forces with germs and argued that the English and Canadians should use bacterial warfare against the Germans first. Allied civilian and military leaders didn't believe the Germans would use bacterial warfare against civilians and rejected Banting's idea of using biological weapons unless the Germans used the weapon first.

Banting's diary contained vague references to using uranium-235 in building an atomic bomb, suggesting he was aware of the United States Manhattan Project. He believed his work at the National Research Council was important but wanted to serve at the front treating wounded soldiers. However, the government kept refusing to send him overseas, saying his work for the council was more important. Banting never gave up the idea of treating wounded soldiers in Europe and made one last effort to serve in Europe by asking to be a passenger on a Lockheed Hudson bomber being ferried to England from Canada. His request was approved, and Banting was outfitted for cold-weather flying by a local Canadian Air Force supply depot. The Hudson bomber took off from an airfield in Montreal on February 17, 1941, headed for Gander, Newfoundland. Flying from Newfoundland to England in a Hudson bomber was dangerous during winter months because bad weather and mechanical problems could cause planes to crash into the snow or the Atlantic Ocean. Only twenty-five Hudson bombers had made the trip to England when Banting was scheduled to fly. Also, Hudson pilots had little experience flying over the ocean in winter. One Hudson bomber had crashed on takeoff and another had been forced to return because of mechanical problems. The civilian crews had minimal experience with the plane, and few pilots knew how to fly long distances over the ocean. It was a risky undertaking, but Banting wanted to get to Europe.

Plane Crash

On February 20, 1941, Banting's plane took off from Gander, Newfoundland, bound for England. The Hudson bomber was about forty miles north of Gander when an oil cooler malfunctioned, and the pilot had to shut down one engine. He planned to fly the disabled plane back to base on the other engine, but the functioning engine's oil system failed a few minutes later, and the plane was left without power. The pilot jettisoned fuel and ordered the crew to throw everything out of the plane because he was going to make a crash landing on a frozen lake just ahead. The plane came down in a snowstorm, hit the tops of some trees, and smashed into the ground just short of the frozen lake he was trying to reach. Two crew members died in the crash, and Banting was unconscious from a serious head injury and a broken arm when the pilot found him in the back of the plane.[262] The pilot had an injured ankle but went outside anyway to look around and survey their situation. He saw that the plane had crash-landed in several feet of snow, the wind was blowing hard, and it was freezing outside. The pilot returned to the plane, turned off the lights to save electrical power, and went to the back of the plane to check on Banting, who was slipping in and out of consciousness.

Banting was incoherent and mumbled something the pilot could not understand, so he wrapped him in blankets and settled down to wait for daylight. In the morning, the pilot decided to go looking for help; he fashioned snowshoes out of tape and map boards, covered Banting with blankets to keep him warm, and set off toward what he thought were lights or a cabin. After hiking through deep snow for several miles, the pilot found nothing and returned to the plane that evening to find that Banting had climbed out of the plane, fell into the snow, and died of exposure. The pilot moved Banting's body back into the plane to await rescue.

Rescuers began searching for the lost plane on February 21 but were unable to see it because the fuselage was covered in snow. The pilot decided to scatter dark powdered aluminum around the plane after he saw a search plane fly over and ignore him. Later, another plane saw the dark streaks of powdered aluminum in the snow and reported the downed plane to authorities. A few hours later, another plane flew low over the aircraft, dropped provisions, and sent a message to trappers living nearby, who came to rescue the pilot and collect the dead bodies. On March 3, 1941, Banting's funeral procession made its way through Toronto followed by an RCAF pipe band. Banting was forty-nine years old and famous when he died.[263]

Chapter 12

---- ✦ ----

PENICILLIN:
ALEXANDER FLEMING

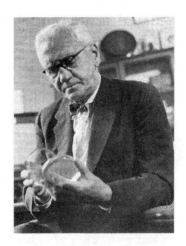

Alexander Fleming recognized that penicillin could kill germs when he saw that one of his culture plates had become contaminated with an unknown mold that inhibited the growth of bacteria. He grew the mold in beef broth and found that the liquid extracted from the mold killed germs causing scarlet fever, pneumonia, gonorrhea, meningitis, diphtheria, and strep throat. Fleming published his findings in the *British Journal of Experimental Pathology* in 1929 and continued trying to purify and manufacture the antibiotic for years with limited success. In 1940, he saw an article in *The Lancet* entitled "Penicillin as a Chemotherapeutic Agent," authored by research scientists at the William Dunn School of Pathology at Oxford University. The Oxford group had discovered how to produce penicillin in larger quantities, successfully tested the antibiotic on animals, and showed that it halted the growth of staphylococcal infection in a human patient. Fleming, Florey, and Chain shared the Nobel Prize for their work on penicillin. Their discovery saved millions of lives.

Alexander Fleming was born on August 6, 1881, near Darvel, England. Fleming attended a local school where he learned reading, writing, arithmetic, and history. In 1894, he enrolled at Kilmarnock Academy to study English, Latin, German, Greek, history, geography, algebra, geometry, trigonometry, chemistry, physics, biology, bookkeeping, and shorthand.[264] In 1895, Fleming entered the Polytechnic-Regent Street in London, where he earned excellent grades and graduated in 1899. He joined the army after graduation and was stationed with the Scottish Regiment in London. While serving with the regiment, Fleming became interested in medicine and enrolled at St. Mary's Hospital Medical School in 1901.[265]

He was an outstanding medical student and got along well with his peers. Fleming studied chemistry, physics, biology, physiology, histology, pharmacology, and anatomy in medical school and spent hours in the dissecting room learning the structure and function of the human body. Medical students accompanied doctors on hospital rounds during their second year to gain experience. Fleming passed his medical qualifying examination in July 1906. He was encouraged to apply for a teaching position at St. Mary's Hospital because the school's rifle team wanted Fleming to join them since he was an excellent shot. St. Mary's Medical School offered Fleming a position in the Inoculation Department and he accepted.[266]

St. Mary's Hospital

At first, Fleming was ambivalent about his job in the bacteriology wing of the Inoculation Department because he wanted to be a surgeon; but after a few months, he became interested in research and spent the next forty-nine years at St. Mary's Hospital. Almroth Wright, head of the Inoculation Department, was an inspiring lecturer and charismatic leader with an abrasive personality, who believed medicine needed to be based on scientific research rather than theory. Fleming began studying acne in the Inoculation Department, isolated the bacillus responsible for the disease, and developed a vaccine that gave immunity to a majority of patients. He took a position as a casualty house surgeon to gain practical experience in operating and passed the exam to become a Fellow of the Royal College of Surgeons. He now had to decide whether to do research or practice surgery. Fleming decided that pursuing research meant he might be able to cure an important disease, so he stayed with Wright to do medical research.

Wright believed immunology was the best way to handle diseases and doubted that antiseptics would be effective because they often caused damage to healthy cells. He received samples of salvarsan from Paul Ehrlich, who had developed the drug as an effective treatment for syphilis. Ehrlich found that salvarsan killed syphilis spirochetes when given intravenously to infected persons, and Fleming was ordered to test the drug to verify Ehrlich's claim.[267] He found that the drug worked well and published his results in *The Lancet* in an article titled "The Use of Salvarsan in the Treatment of Syphilis." Following the publication of the article, Fleming developed a lucrative private practice treating syphilis and seemed destined to become a specialist in handling sexually transmitted diseases. An advance in the diagnosis of syphilis occurred when August von Wassermann developed a reliable test for the disease in 1906, but it required a fairly large sample of blood from the patient. Fleming wanted to develop a test that used only a small amount of blood to test for syphilis.

Wassermann Test

Fleming modified Wassermann's test so it worked with the amount of blood serum obtained from a finger prick. However, when Fleming's test was used by other doctors, it missed about one-quarter of syphilis infections. Fleming studied the procedures used by other physicians and concluded they had neglected to wash the serum with saline before performing the Wassermann test. He showed that doctors who followed his procedures carefully found his modified test to be accurate.

Fleming resigned from the Scottish Regiment in 1914 to devote full-time to his research. Four months later, World War I broke out in Europe. The Scottish Regiment suffered terrible losses at the Battle of Messines in 1917 in Belgium, and if Fleming had been with the regiment, the discovery of antibiotics could have been delayed for years. Wright was appointed a lieutenant colonel in the Royal Army Medical Corps and sent to France to establish a laboratory for studying wound infections among English soldiers. He took his team to France, including Fleming, who was commissioned a lieutenant in the British Army.[268] Wright convinced the British military to inoculate all soldiers against typhoid, and St. Mary's Hospital helped produce ten million doses of typhoid vaccine during the war. Because of vaccination, the Allies lost only twelve hundred men to typhoid during the war rather than the one hundred twenty thousand expected to die from the disease had the soldiers not been vaccinated. Fleming was assigned the task of studying battlefield infections by Wright.

Battlefield Infections

He took swabs from patients' wounds before and after surgery, collected bullets removed from wounded soldiers, gathered shell fragments extracted from wounds, cut parts from wounded soldiers' uniforms, and accumulated tissue and bone fragments from surgical wards for study. Fleming found that over 90 percent of the samples taken from new uniforms contained bacteria that caused gangrene. He also found tetanus, streptococcus, and staphylococcus bacteria on the new clothing. Fleming concluded that infectious organisms from uniforms entered the soldiers' wounds along with the bullet or shell fragment, and the germs grew in dead tissue without oxygen. Fleming concluded that antiseptics were being absorbed by bandages and dead tissue on the surface of the wound while bacteria deeper in the wound were unaffected, continued to multiply, and killed patients. His article in *The Lancet* was the first comprehensive study of wound infections ever published. Fleming's next assignment involved treating sexually transmitted diseases in military hospitals.

Based on his expertise in diagnosing and treating sexually transmitted diseases, Fleming was ordered back to England to establish venereal disease treatment facilities at major military hospitals. He was appointed chief pathologist for all venereal disease treatment facilities in England. His job was to study sexually transmitted diseases and distribute salvarsan to clinics and hospitals. In 1917, Fleming was appointed bacteriologist at a military hospital treating bone fractures. His earlier work on wound infections helped Fleming design treatments that reduced gangrene among these patients. In 1918, the influenza pandemic created additional stress on military physicians and killed thousands of young soldiers. Fleming found that most deaths during the pandemic were caused by secondary infections such as pneumonia rather than influenza itself. In 1919, he was released from the military and returned to St. Mary's Hospital. Fleming's work during the war had enhanced his medical reputation; he was considered the world's leading expert on wound infections.[269]

For the first time in years, Fleming was able to work a normal eight-hour day rather than having to work around the clock treating wounded patients. He had married Sarah McElroy, a nurse he met during the war, and they established a home in Chelsea where they settled into a comfortable married routine. Fleming was made assistant director of the Inoculation Department. He began studying bactericides and searching for a better antiseptic to keep patients free of infections following surgery. He found that human body fluids have natural antibacterial qualities and decided to study them in detail.

Antibacterial Mucus

In November 1921, Fleming was suffering from a cold and decided to culture some of the mucus from his nose to see what happened. A few days later, he inspected the culture and found it covered with yellow colonies of bacteria except around the area where Fleming had placed mucus from his nose. Something in his mucus was killing bacteria in the petri dish, and he wanted to discover how it worked. Fleming placed some of the bacteria from the petri dish in a saline solution and added more of his nasal mucus. In a few minutes, the solution was clear—the mucus had somehow dissolved the bacteria. Fleming didn't understand what was happening, so he decided to see if mucus would kill other types of bacteria. He speculated that he was dealing with natural human immunity to bacteria and set out to discover how many different types of bacteria might be susceptible to nasal mucus. Fleming found that nasal mucus killed only staphylococci bacteria, so it was not a very useful antiseptic.

He decided to try nasal mucus from other people to make certain there was nothing unique about the mucus from his nose. Fleming found the same results using mucus from other people and decided to see if other body fluids had a similar ability to kill staphylococci bacteria. He collected tears, saliva, sputum, blood serum, and plasma to test as bacterial antiseptics. Fleming found that these body fluids had the ability to dissolve staphylococci bacteria. Also, skin, mucus membranes, internal organs, hair, and fingernails produced the same antibacterial effect. Finally, he examined tissue from rabbits, guinea pigs, and dogs and discovered these animals' body fluids dissolved staphylococci bacteria as well although the effect was stronger in fluid from some animals compared with others. Fleming concluded that body fluids from many animals contain a substance that kills staphylococci bacteria, and he wanted to understand what it was and how it worked.

Fleming was convinced he had discovered something important, but because he was not a chemist, he had no idea what substance he was studying or how it worked. He named the antibacterial substance "lysozyme" and found that temperatures over seventy degrees Centigrade (158 degrees Fahrenheit) destroyed lysozyme's ability to kill staphylococci bacteria. Fleming also showed that lysozyme was precipitated by alcohol and acetone, chemicals that precipitate proteins. He believed he was working with an enzyme because the liquids seemed to dissolve bacteria. Fleming wondered if he had discovered a new antiseptic. However, since only a few strains of staphylococci, streptococci, and pneumococci were affected, he concluded that the antiseptic would be of limited use. Nevertheless, it was an advance in understanding the human immunology system. Fleming reported his findings to the local Medical Research Club in December 1921. He continued working with lysozyme and found that after repeated exposure, germs became resistant—a problem that has plagued antibiotics for years. This early work with lysozyme prepared Fleming to notice that a mold that fell on one of his bacterial cultures killed bacteria, leading to the discovery of penicillin.

Penicillin

He first saw penicillin's ability to destroy bacteria on September 3, 1928, when Fleming returned from a vacation. He preserved the original culture plate contaminated with the mold that killed bacteria, showing he understood the importance of the observation immediately.[270] Fleming realized he had discovered a new antibiotic and wanted to learn how to produce a supply of what he called "mold juice," which was a filtrate of the broth in which he grew the mold. The mold juice he prepared was impure, but adequate for doing preliminary research because he was not using animal subjects to test the effectiveness of what later turned out to be the antibiotic he called penicillin. Fleming tried different media for growing the mold and found that ordinary meat broth produced good results.

His next step was to find the best temperature and interval for growing the mold. Trial and error testing showed that room temperature and about five days were optimum for producing full-strength mold juice. After Fleming discovered how to grow the mold in liquid broth, he made grooves across the jelly in a petri dish and filled the grooves with liquid mold extract. Once the mixture of broth and mold extract solidified, Fleming used a platinum wire to spread bacterial cultures at right angles to the grooves he had made in the petri dish and incubated the mixture at body temperature, which he found was best for growing bacteria. Fleming saw that the mold juice (penicillin) diffused a short distance on each side of the grooves had created an inhibition zone where bacteria sensitive to penicillin would not grow. He measured the size of each inhibition zone around the penicillin groove and used the measurement as a rough indicator of how sensitive a particular bacterium was to penicillin. Fleming found that penicillin killed gram-positive bacteria.

Gram-Positive Bacteria

Fleming tested many bacteria to see which were killed by penicillin and found that the antibiotic inhibits the growth of gram-positive pathogens, which are germs that stain with purple dye. Gram-positive bacteria include the germs that cause scarlet fever, pneumonia, gonorrhea, meningitis, diphtheria, and strep throat.[271] Fleming also showed that penicillin was more effective at killing bacteria than carbolic acid and didn't harm healthy tissue or blood cells. At first, Fleming believed he had found the perfect antibiotic; but when he mixed penicillin with blood serum, the antibiotic seemed to lose its effectiveness, and he began to wonder if it would work in human patients at all.

Fleming decided he should know what mold he was using to produce his mold juice and contacted C. J. La Touche, who was studying the effect of molds on asthmatic patients. After a little research, La Touche told Fleming he was working with *Penicillium rubrum*. However, Fleming later discovered that his mold was actually *Penicillium notatum*. He called the mold juice *penicillin* and set out to learn whether the mold he was using was unique or if other molds would also kill bacteria. In the process of searching for other germ-killing molds, Fleming developed one of the first screening programs to find antibiotics that kill bacteria. He collected samples from moldy jam, cheese, fruits, and other substances to test their ability to inhibit bacterial growth. Fleming found that his original mold was the only one with the ability to kill bacteria. He also wanted to understand the chemical properties of penicillin and how to produce it in large quantities. But Fleming was no chemist, so he went looking for someone to help him with the analysis. He enlisted Frederick Ridley and Stuart Craddock to help develop a method of producing penicillin in larger quantities and analyze its chemical composition.

Attempts to Manufacture Penicillin

Ridley and Craddock began by growing the mold in five-liter containers at room temperature. After a few days, the containers developed a fluffy white mass floating on the surface of the nutrient fluid. After a few more days, the mold they were growing developed a yellow color, and they found it would kill bacteria. Liquid from the yellow mold was filtered under pressure through cheesecloth, paper, and asbestos pads to produce a moderately pure form of liquid penicillin. They placed the filtered penicillin in a vacuum flask and concentrated it by heating and removing the gas with a vacuum pump. This procedure generated a viscous mixture of penicillin and impurities that they used for further study.

Fleming believed penicillin was an enzyme, but Ridley and Craddock thought he was wrong. If it were an enzyme, the viscous mixture should dissolve in water but not alcohol. However, when they added alcohol to the penicillin mixture, it dissolved and killed bacteria when diluted to concentrations of 1 to 3,000. Dissolving the penicillin in alcohol effectively separated protein from nonprotein materials, and they discovered to their surprise that the active ingredient in penicillin was something in the liquid. Finding that penicillin dissolved in alcohol opened new manufacturing options because it's easier to evaporate alcohol than water at low temperatures. However, the penicillin Ridley and Craddock produced was impure and lost its ability to kill bacteria in just a few days at room temperature. They found that maintaining a pH value of 6.5 (slightly basic) prolonged the ability of penicillin to kill bacteria for several weeks, so they were able to produce and store enough antibiotic for use in animal studies.

Clinical Effects in Animals

Fleming decided he was ready to begin exploring the clinical effects of penicillin, and Craddock volunteered to ingest penicillin grown in milk. He suffered no ill effects, so they concluded it was not toxic to human beings when taken orally.[272] A dangerous initial test. Today, experimental penicillin would have been tested on animals first rather than a human subject. Fleming next treated a patient who had a streptococcal infection in the gut, but the oral dose of penicillin had no effect on his infection. A patient with an infected stump following an amputation was tested after that, but the topical application of penicillin produced similar poor results.

Fleming concluded that oral and topical application of penicillin wouldn't work and began looking for an alternate way to administer the drug. He reasoned that penicillin was not able to penetrate into the body through oral or topical application and that it needed to be injected into a muscle or the bloodstream to produce an antibacterial effect. Fleming decided to publish his work on penicillin in the *British Journal of Experimental Pathology* in 1929.

Prior Claims

Following the publication of Fleming's paper, many other scientists claimed they had noted that penicillin kills bacteria before Fleming; but since these claims were unsubstantiated, they were ignored by medical authorities. Fleming believed other physicians probably had noticed that molds kill bacteria and doctors had recommended using molds to treat infections since Galen's time, but those earlier physicians had not grown quantities of the mold, separated the active part of the mold from its impurities, produced an antibiotic, and proved it would actually kill bacteria. The only priority claim that came close to Fleming's was made by Andre D. Gratia at the University of Liege. Gratia had been studying the antibacterial action of a green mold that seemed to inhibit the growth of anthrax, but fell ill, lost his antibiotic mold culture, and was not able to reproduce it. Gratia told Fleming about his work and asked for recognition, but made clear he was not claiming priority for Fleming's discovery of penicillin.

First Success with Penicillin

Craddock and Ridley left the St. Mary's bacteriological laboratory to pursue their own research in 1930, and Fleming was again left alone to develop and test penicillin. In 1933, he was able to successfully treat an infected patient using penicillin. His assistant, Keith Rogers, developed an eye infection and was worried he could not compete in a shooting contest the following weekend, but Fleming said he could help. He put some yellow penicillin fluid in Rogers's eye, telling him it would clear up the infection in time for the shooting match.[273] The penicillin worked, and Rogers was probably the first patient treated successfully with penicillin applied locally to his eye.

Fleming had difficulty finding suitable patients and producing a sufficient supply of penicillin at the same time because his penicillin only remained effective for a few days, and he had difficulty finding a proper patient during that short interval. Once his penicillin became ineffective, it took several days to make a new batch. Fleming recognized that until he had clear evidence that penicillin was effective in treating infected human patients, he would not be able to find a pharmaceutical company willing to manufacture the antibiotic in large quantities. Meanwhile, other scientists were getting interested in studying penicillin.

Biochemistry of Penicillin

Harold Raistrick and Reginald Lovell began studying chemically active molds after reading Fleming's article about penicillin. Their assistant called Fleming to find out what was the best medium for growing the mold, and he was happy to help. However, Raistrick and Lovell were unable to purify the penicillin they produced and gave up their research program. When he learned of their failure, Fleming became concerned that he would never be able to purify penicillin and prove it was an effective antibiotic. He returned to studying penicillin in 1934 when Lewis Holt, a chemist, joined the St. Mary's Hospital staff. Fleming showed Holt his work on penicillin and suggested they jointly try to understand the chemistry of penicillin. Holt agreed to work with Fleming to purify and study the antibiotic.

Holt tried extracting the active ingredient in liquid penicillin using acidic amyl acetate and found that the procedure worked. He was able to recover the active ingredient in penicillin from the acidic amyl acetate solution by using an alkaline aqueous solution of sodium bicarbonate.[274] This procedure also removed many of the impurities in the mold extract and produced an almost pure form of penicillin. Unfortunately, Holt didn't realize that his procedure for producing nearly pure penicillin was a success and abandoned the project without sharing his results with Fleming—an early missed opportunity. Fleming continued working on penicillin for the next several years, studying the effect of acidity on the shelf life of penicillin, and trying to extend the interval penicillin remained effective by storing it in different containers under seal. He also grew the mold on paper and showed that it produced an effective antibiotic. Fleming studied how bacteria develop resistance to penicillin but was distracted from studying it further when he received a sample of a new antibiotic called sulfanilamide from a German manufacturer.

Sulfanilamide

Sulfanilamide, or "sulfa" as the drug came to be called, was originally developed by Gerhard Domagk at the I. G. Farben Bayer plant in Dusseldorf, Germany. The drug offered an effective treatment for pneumonia, meningitis, scarlet fever, and puerperal fever. Domagk won the Nobel Prize for his discovery in 1939. Although sulfa was effective in killing bacteria, it produced significant side effects, including skin rash, vomiting, and on rare occasions, suppression of white blood cell production, reducing the ability of the body to fight off infections. Fleming began studying sulfa in 1939. He discovered that bacteria killed by sulfa drug consume a nutrient chemically similar to sulfonamide and mistakenly take up the sulfa drug instead, starving themselves in the process. Meanwhile, a medical team at Oxford University became interested in Fleming's reports on penicillin and began working on purifying and producing the antibiotic in larger quantities.

The Oxford Group

In August of 1940, as the German bombing of London was beginning, Fleming opened his copy of The Lancet and saw an article entitled "Penicillin as a Chemotherapeutic Agent," authored by scientists working at the William Dunn School of Pathology at Oxford University. The article concluded that penicillin had a therapeutic potential, which encouraged Fleming to visit Oxford and discuss their research results. He arrived at

Oxford University on September 2, 1940, and was shown around their laboratory and told what the team was doing. The Oxford group had begun their work in 1938 and set out to discover how to produce a large supply of the antibiotic, overcome its tendency to lose effectiveness, understand its biochemistry, and test the drug's clinical application in treating human infections.

In 1940, they decided to develop a standard method of measuring the efficacy of penicillin so they could report their results accurately. The Oxford team tried several methods and settled on using a standard petri dish containing agar into which six short lengths of glass tubing filled with penicillin solution were inserted. The Oxford team spread bacteria on the agar in the petri dish and incubated the dish while the penicillin diffused from the glass tubes. By measuring the diameter of the penicillin circle at the ends of the glass tubes where it had killed bacteria, the Oxford team was able to estimate the effectiveness of the penicillin solution at killing different bacteria. They decided to use the amount of penicillin contained in one centimeter of solution as their standard dose. Once they established a standard way of measuring the effectiveness of penicillin and a standard unit of the antibiotic, the Oxford team set about isolating penicillin from the liquid produced by fermenting mold.

They dissolved the penicillin liquid in ether and found they had difficulty extracting it afterward. They finally tried extracting penicillin from the ether by using slightly alkaline water, and the process worked, as it had for Holt years earlier. Also, most impurities were removed from the penicillin by the extraction process. The Oxford team found that the penicillin they produced was stable for several months when stored at zero degrees Centigrade and could be freeze-dried to make it last even longer. By 1940, the Oxford team had produced over one hundred milligrams of brown powdered penicillin for use in clinical trials on animals. The penicillin powder was still impure, but they decided it was safe to use on animals to determine if the drug was toxic. The Oxford team injected penicillin into two mice and concluded it was probably harmless. They were now prepared to determine if penicillin killed bacteria in animals. On May 25, 1940, while British troops were being evacuated from Dunkirk, they infected eight mice with streptococci bacteria. Two of the mice were given one ten-milligram dose of penicillin by injection, two other mice received five milligrams of penicillin injected on four separate occasions over ten hours, and the other four mice were left untreated. The four untreated mice died the next day while the four mice treated with different doses of penicillin remained alive and healthy. The Oxford team concluded in their article that penicillin kills bacteria in living animals and was probably safe for use in humans.

Fleming returned from Oxford with a sample of the best penicillin the team had produced and a clear understanding of how they manufactured the drug. He believed that growing penicillin from mold was inefficient, and a new method was needed so it could be manufactured in larger quantities. The Oxford group established a facility in their laboratory to produce enough penicillin to conduct clinical trials on humans. By January 1941, they had an adequate supply of penicillin to treat one patient and asked a doctor at Radcliffe Infirmary to find a dying patient who would agree to receive an injection of penicillin because he or she had nothing to lose. They found a woman dying of breast cancer who agreed to try the new antibiotic. After receiving an injection of penicillin, she reported a metallic taste in her mouth and developed a temperature, probably caused by impurities in the drug. Other than those minor side effects, the penicillin injection appeared safe for use on healthy patients, so the Oxford team set about planning a clinical trial on an infected human patient.

First Penicillin Cure

They discovered that injecting penicillin into an intravenous drip of saline was an effective way to deliver the antibiotic into the human bloodstream. Albert Alexander, a forty-three-year-old policeman, volunteered to be their first patient.[275] He had become infected with staphylococcal bacteria after he scratched his face on a rose thorn. Albert had nothing to lose by taking penicillin because he was dying of a bacterial infection. On February 12, 1941, he was administered two hundred milligrams of penicillin and then given three hundred milligrams of penicillin every three hours afterward.

Penicillin was in such short supply that his urine was collected, the penicillin separated from it, and reused. After five days, Alexander was recovering from his infection, but the supply of penicillin ran out and he eventually died. The Oxford team decided to test the drug on children with localized infections because they would require less penicillin for treatment, and the team could test the antibiotic on more patients. They treated children with a variety of infections over the next few weeks and found that penicillin cured them all. The Oxford team published their results in August 1941 in *The Lancet*.

They traveled to America after the clinical trials were finished, hoping to find a US pharmaceutical company willing to manufacture penicillin since the British pharmaceutical industry was busy producing vaccines and medicines for the war effort and had neither the time nor the money to experiment with manufacturing a new antibiotic. The Rockefeller Foundation gave the Oxford team $6,000 to cover their expenses during the US trip. Merck, Squibb, Pfizer, and Lederle all agreed to produce penicillin for the US government after discussing the Oxford team's results. In England, Kemball Bishop began producing penicillin on a small scale for use in clinical trials, but there was little interest among English pharmaceutical firms in manufacturing large quantities of penicillin. The English government was totally unprepared to handle the huge demand for penicillin that developed after it became clear the drug was effective in killing infections. Fleming met with the British Ministry of Supply on September 25, 1942, to urge the government to make a stronger effort to produce penicillin in England. The Imperial Chemical Industries and Parke-Davis began working on producing penicillin in England, but they were far behind the US pharmaceutical companies by that time and were short of staff and money as well.

Producing Penicillin

Production of penicillin rose dramatically over the next few years, especially in the US. In 1942, the only penicillin available was produced in England at Oxford University. By 1943, enough penicillin was being produced in the

US to begin running clinical trials on the battlefields of Europe and in the Pacific. The effects were dramatic; soldiers who would have lost limbs to serious infections were cured in a few days and eventually returned to fight. The military decided they would use their limited supplies of penicillin to treat sexually transmitted diseases so these soldiers could return to the battlefield immediately rather than having to wait weeks for a wound to heal. Large supplies of penicillin began arriving from America in late 1943, so the drug could be used for treating both sexually transmitted diseases and war wounds from that point forward. Penicillin was released for civilian use late in 1943.

Fleming and the Oxford team both believed they had discovered penicillin, and the disagreement produced hard feelings on both sides. The Oxford team discouraged contacts with the press but suspected that Fleming was secretly advancing his claim to the discovery of penicillin by holding private discussions with reporters. Based on his discovery of penicillin, Fleming was elected a fellow of the Royal Society on March 18, 1943, and was listed as the discoverer of penicillin by the press. He appeared on the cover of *Time* magazine in May 1944 and received $2,720 in contributions from US readers of the magazine. Fleming used the funds for research and shared credit with the Oxford group for their work in perfecting the purification of penicillin and showing it was clinically effective in killing infections among humans, but they were jealous of Fleming's greater fame.

After the war, Fleming toured America and was hailed as the discoverer of penicillin. He was surprised to find that the United States appreciated his work more than the British. Fleming was given a banquet at the Waldorf Hotel, and the American Association of Penicillin Producers gave him a check for $100,000, which he donated to the St. Mary's Inoculation Department to support basic research. The American trip started a new phase in Fleming's life; he became a world ambassador for penicillin. After returning to England, he set off for Paris as a guest of the French government to discuss penicillin supplies with authorities in that country. The French government wanted to ensure the country would receive a supply of penicillin because they were unable to manufacture it themselves and hoped that Fleming would help them import the drug from America. He also went to Italy, met the pope, and made the rounds of British military hospitals before flying to Denmark and Sweden.

Nobel Prize

On October 25, 1945, Alexander Fleming of St. Mary's Hospital and Howard Florey and Ernst Chain of Oxford University were awarded the Nobel Prize in medicine for their discovery and development of penicillin.[276] Fleming was awarded half the prize for his discovery of penicillin, and Florey and Chain were jointly given the other half of the prize for their work on purifying penicillin and showing that it was clinically effective in humans. Fleming went to Sweden to receive the award and continued his world travels for the remainder of his life as the discoverer of penicillin. He received honors and awards from countries on both sides of the Iron Curtain but had trouble traveling to Soviet-dominated areas. His feelings about the attention were mixed, relishing the recognition but finding that large formal gatherings made him uncomfortable. Fleming tolerated the travel and attention out of a sense of duty to British science and the importance he attached to promoting penicillin around the world, but he didn't enjoy the fame.

Fleming was inundated with requests from young scientists who wanted to work with him, but there were few posts available at St. Mary's Hospital although he was willing to have them come if they could support themselves or simply needed advice. These young scientists were often disappointed; they expected Fleming to give them exciting research ideas to pursue, but he was so busy with travel and administrative duties he had little time for discussing or thinking about research. He continued working in the field of bacteriology; but his research took second place to public appearances, travel, and administrative duties as director of the Institute of Therapeutic Research at St. Mary's Hospital. Fleming was an efficient administrator, but postponed decisions when possible, creating problems for his staff.

When the British National Health Service was established after the war, many doctors opposed nationalizing medical care because they feared a loss of status and income. No matter what doctors thought of the new medical service, they had to accept it once the National Health Service was authorized by law. Fleming was forced to retire from his post as a professor of bacteriology in 1948 when he turned sixty-seven, and his retirement was marred by his wife's declining health. Sareen Fleming fell ill in 1948; her health declined rapidly, and she died on October 8, 1949.

Fleming eventually married Dr. Amalia Voureka, a member of the Inoculation Department who worked in his laboratory. She had been involved in the Greek resistance during the war, helping Greek and British soldiers escape from the country. She was arrested by the German occupation forces and held in Averof Prison for six months during the war. At the end of the war, she applied for a British Council scholarship to study in London at St. Mary's Hospital. When her scholarship ended, Fleming offered her a research scholarship so she could continue assisting him, which she accepted. Amalia was eventually appointed head of bacteriology at Evangelismos Hospital in Greece and left London. Fleming followed her to Greece in 1952 and, on his last night in the country, proposed marriage. Amalia accepted, and after their wedding in 1953, they traveled to Cuba and the United States on their honeymoon.[277] When they returned to St. Mary's Hospital, many members of the staff were scandalized by their thirty-one-year age difference and the fact that she was considered arrogant by many in the hospital.

Last Days

Fleming resigned as director of the institute and retired in January 1955. He contracted influenza in February of that year and never fully recovered. On March 10, he was given an antithyroid inoculation in preparation for a trip to Turkey and Greece. The next day, he felt sick, experienced pain in his chest, and vomited. Amalia called his physician and told him it was probably not serious, but she would like the doctor to see her husband later that day. Fleming told Amalia he didn't believe he was having heart problems just a few minutes before he suffered a severe heart attack and died on March 11, 1955.[278] His ashes were placed in a crypt at St. Paul's Cathedral near such British greats as Lord Nelson and the Duke of Wellington.

Chapter 13

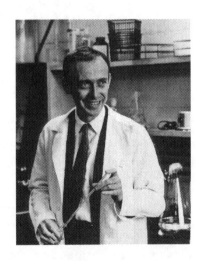

STRUCTURE OF DNA: JAMES WATSON

J ames Watson was working in the Cavendish Laboratory at Cambridge, England, when he met Francis Crick. They jointly decided to study the structure of DNA and were aided by X-ray diffraction photographs produced by Rosalind Franklin and Maurice Wilkins. Watson and Crick discovered the structure of DNA by building physical models and comparing their structure with measurements taken from X-ray diffraction photographs. They decided to construct the simplest model they could imagine, believing that was their best strategy. Early models didn't produce the proper angles and distances required by the X-ray diffraction photographs, but Watson eventually built a DNA model he believed was accurate. After measuring several angles and distances to verify that his model satisfied the X-ray data and laws of chemistry, Watson and Crick showed their work to Maurice Wilkins. Wilkins confirmed that measurements from his X-ray diffraction photographs were consistent with Watson and Crick's model. Francis Crick, James Watson, and Maurice Wilkins were awarded the Nobel Prize in Physiology or Medicine in 1962 "for their discoveries concerning the molecular structure of nucleic acids and its significance for information transfer in living material."

James Watson was born on April 6, 1928, in Chicago, Illinois. He attended Horace Mann Grammar School and South Shore High School. Watson enrolled in the University of Chicago at fifteen. He graduated in 1947 and went to Indiana University for his PhD.[279] After earning his doctorate, Watson spent a year as a postdoctoral fellow at Copenhagen University studying enzyme metabolism and got interested in understanding the structure of DNA. He wanted to learn about X-ray diffraction but couldn't do that in Copenhagen, so he decided to move to England and work at Cambridge University in the Cavendish Laboratory.

Cavendish Laboratory

The Fellowship Board in Washington refused to give Watson permission to move his fellowship to England, but he had saved money from earlier fellowships and had funds to support himself for a year without a government fellowship. In 1951, he began working in the Cavendish Laboratory at Cambridge, where he planned to learn X-ray diffraction and study the three-dimensional structure of proteins. Watson met Francis Crick, a former physicist student who was working on a PhD in biology at Cambridge, found they had similar interests and decided to work together studying the structure of DNA.[280] At that time, Linus Pauling in America and Maurice Wilkins in England were the leading researchers trying to understand the molecular structure of DNA. Wilkins was working with Rosalind Franklin, who was doing X-ray diffraction studies in his laboratory.

X-ray Diffraction

Rosalind Franklin and Maurice Wilkins produced the X-ray diffraction photographs that allowed Watson and Crick to build a double helix model of DNA and verify it was correct.[281] Franklin died of cancer in 1958, so she was denied a chance to share the 1962 Nobel Prize in Physiology or Medicine awarded to Watson, Crick, and Wilkins. Only living scientists can receive the award. Watson said Franklin's X-ray photographs played a large role in their discovery of DNA's structure and receiving the Nobel Prize. Sir Lawrence Bragg, director of the Cavendish Laboratory, first showed that X-rays are diffracted in unique ways based on the structure of the crystals employed. His work led to the development of X-ray crystallography. Bragg was awarded the Nobel Prize for his work.

Crick was studying the structure of proteins at Cambridge and had the ability to understand other people's experimental work quickly and develop a plausible theory of what their data meant. His ability made other scientists at Cambridge wary because they feared he might borrow their ideas and publish them in his own theoretical articles. Before Watson arrived, Crick had not spent much time working on DNA, but his experience studying the structure of proteins was critical when they began working together. Crick had avoided studying the structure of DNA before Watson joined him at Cavendish because that research area was considered the personal domain of Maurice Wilkins. This made no difference to an ambitious young American scientist such as Watson, but polite English researchers didn't poach in their friend's research fields; Wilkins had been studying the structure of DNA for years, and it was "his" area.

Maurice Wilkins

Wilkins had been using X-ray diffraction to study DNA for years, and Crick felt it would not be fair to begin working on the same problem using similar procedures after Wilkins had spent so much time and effort trying to understand the structure of DNA. The issue was further complicated because Wilkins had brought Rosalind Franklin to King's College London as his assistant to help him with X-ray diffraction research. But when she arrived, Franklin announced that studying the X-ray diffraction of DNA was her exclusive domain, and she didn't intend to be Wilkins's assistant. She wanted an equal share of the credit for any important discovery they made. Wilkins wanted her to act as his assistant or leave King's College London, but Franklin insisted she had to be Wilkins's equal partner at King's College and would not agree to leave. He was unsure how to handle this difficult situation. To make matters worse, Linus Pauling at Caltech in California had asked Wilkins to send him a copy of the crystalline DNA X-ray photographs produced by Rosalind Franklin so he could study them personally. After some delay, Wilkins finally told Pauling he wanted to study the photographs in more detail himself before he released them publicly and refused to send any photographs to California. Watson grew interested in studying DNA after he heard a lecture on the subject given by Wilkins in Italy.

Interest in DNA

Watson became interested in studying the molecular structure of DNA using X-ray diffraction after listening to a presentation on the subject by Wilkins at a conference in Naples, Italy, in 1951. Salvador Luria, Watson's supervisor in Copenhagen, had suggested earlier that solving the working of genetics might be accomplished by looking at the chemical structure of DNA to discover how genes are duplicated. Luria said he believed DNA was the essential part of a gene and told Watson that little was known of its structure, so that was a good research area to explore. Most biochemists believed DNA was a large acid composed of smaller acids, but its basic structure and how it might work was a mystery. Watson was interested in understanding DNA, but he had little idea how to proceed until he heard Wilkins describe his work on X-ray diffraction and DNA.

Making X-ray diffraction photographs of DNA seemed to Watson an excellent way to study the molecular structure of genes. During his presentation, Wilkins said X-ray diffraction photographs suggested DNA might be a crystalline substance, and when the structure of DNA was understood, biologists would be able to understand how genes replicate, which was exactly what Watson wanted to know. Watson knew that if a gene were a crystal, it should have a regular structure that could be understood in a simple way by developing a molecular model of its structure. He decided to meet Wilkins and discuss joining his laboratory, but couldn't find him at the conference. The next day, his sister joined Watson in Naples, and they arranged to meet Wilkins for lunch. However, Wilkins didn't seem interested in discussing X-ray diffraction with Watson, so he concluded his future probably didn't involve working with Watkins. He decided to stay at Cavendish Laboratory and work on X-ray diffraction with Crick rather than trying to join Wilkins in London. They had a serious competitor in America named Linus Pauling.

Linus Pauling

Watson discovered that Linus Pauling had solved the structure of proteins by playing around with building simple molecular models, which suggested to him that the same method might be a fruitful way to proceed with studying the structure of DNA.[282] Pauling had recently shown that protein was an alpha-helix, which he said was simple and beautiful. Scientists trained in structural chemistry believed Pauling had discovered something important and were impressed with his work. Watson soon realized that if he wanted to study the structure of DNA using X-ray diffraction, he would need to know how to produce, understand, and interpret X-ray diffraction photographs. He made an appointment with Max Perutz (who won the Nobel Prize in Chemistry for his work on the structure of hemoglobin), explained what he wanted to do, and asked him for advice about how to proceed. Perutz told Watson he should have no problem understanding X-ray diffraction if he studied basic crystallography because the field was not that complex. Watson was encouraged and decided to discuss the issue with Crick and see what his partner thought of modeling DNA.

When Watson told Crick about Pauling's modeling work on the structure of proteins, his friend immediately concluded that the same technique would work to discover the molecular structure of DNA. Crick told Watson he was interested in understanding the structure of DNA, but needed to finish his dissertation because Bragg was pressuring him to complete his degree and leave. However, Crick said he was willing to work with Watson on the molecular structure of DNA and teach him the crystallographic facts that could only be acquired by reading esoteric journal articles while he worked on his degree. They agreed to form a partnership to study DNA.

Modeling DNA

Crick told Watson that Pauling's discovery of the alpha-helix structure of proteins was based on the application of common sense rather than a giant leap of logic or a huge creative insight, and they should be able to do the same thing with DNA. Crick believed Pauling had relied mainly on his knowledge of structural chemistry in developing his model of proteins and speculated that Pauling had simply asked himself which atoms must sit next to each other and then used a set of models similar to the Tinkertoys used by preschool children to construct the alpha-helix model of proteins by trial and error. Crick didn't see any fundamental reason why they couldn't use a similar technique to uncover the structure of DNA. Crick said they should ask the Cavendish shop to build the basic components of DNA so they could connect them to form models, play with the models until they hit on the right structure of DNA, and then compare their model with the X-ray diffraction photographs taken by Wilkins and Franklin. Simple in theory, but complicated in reality.

Crick suggested they start by assuming that the molecular structure of DNA was a simple helix because any other structure would be much more complicated. They also agreed to assume DNA was composed of a large number of nucleotides (a molecule containing nitrogen and phosphate) linked together in a simple way, and that the structure of DNA was a simple helix based on sugar phosphates linked in a three-dimensional pattern. They further assumed that the backbone of DNA had identical chemical connections. Crick recalled that Wilkins had said the diameter of a DNA molecule was larger than would be the case if DNA was constructed with only one chain, and therefore it was more likely that the structure of DNA was a compound helix constructed of nucleotides twisted around each other. They also assumed DNA contained four types of nucleotides and that the nucleotides all contained sugar and phosphate components. They believed the differences among the four nucleotides most likely occurred in their nitrogenous bases. Watson and Crick hypothesized that the linkages between nucleotides involved phosphate and sugar groups, which formed a regular backbone for the DNA.

However, to build and test their models, Watson and Crick needed to have access to copies of the X-ray diffraction photographs taken by Wilkins and Franklin because measurements taken from them would limit the possible structures they would consider and tell them if their model was correct. They had already found a reasonably clear X-ray diffraction photograph published by W. T. Astbury a few years before, but they wanted to see the X-ray diffraction photographs of DNA taken by Franklin because those could save them months of work developing models of DNA that didn't fit the latest evidence. The photographs were in the possession of Wilkins, so they had to clear the matter with him. Crick called Wilkins, and he agreed to travel to Cambridge to meet with them and discuss his work.

Double Helix

When Wilkins met with Watson and Crick, he agreed that the structure of DNA was probably a helix, so they might well be on the right track.[283] However, when they outlined their idea of how to proceed, Wilkins said he didn't think that model building was the best way to discover the structure of DNA. Even more troubling for Watson and Crick's plan, Rosalind Franklin had told Wilkins he must not make any more X-ray diffraction photographs of DNA because that was her domain and she didn't want him working in her area. Trying to placate Franklin, Wilkins had given her the rest of the crystalline DNA he had used to make his original photographs; so there was no DNA available for Wilkins, Watson, or Crick to produce more X-ray diffraction photographs. Moreover, Wilkins and Franklin were estranged, and she would not discuss her work with him. Wilkins told Watson and Crick their best tactic would be to wait until Franklin gave a seminar in a few weeks because she would discuss her work before a public audience and they could see the X-ray diffraction photographs then. Watson decided he needed to learn more about crystallography so he could understand Rosalind Franklin's presentation.

To complicate matters even more, Crick had a disagreement with his supervising professor when he learned that Bragg had used one of his ideas in a paper published with Max Perutz without giving Crick credit. Bragg became angry at Crick's suggestion he had stolen the idea and suggested Crick should find another place to work if that was how he felt. Bragg's response created a serious problem for Crick because he desperately needed an adviser and a place to work, and he had already a reputation as a difficult person to supervise so his options were limited. Crick's friends stepped in and calmed Sir Bragg, who agreed to allow Crick to stay if he got to work on his PhD project immediately and stopped working on DNA. Crick was forced to agree. Watson decided to go ahead with the study of X-ray diffraction on his own and hope for the best.

A Mathematical Test for Molecular Models

While working on his thesis, Crick began thinking about a general mathematical way to test molecular models. He worked on the problem for a few days and believed he had discovered the solution. Crick developed the proper equations and discussed them with Bill Cochran, a lecturer in crystallography at Cavendish, who agreed Crick was right. The two decided to publish a short paper on the topic in *Nature* and send a copy to Linus Pauling at Caltech for his comments. Crick now had a solid theoretical publication under his belt, felt more comfortable with his academic position, and decided he could safely work on the structure of DNA with Watson while he finished his thesis. Meanwhile, Franklin's seminar was approaching, and Watson needed to be prepared.

Before attending Franklin's seminar, Watson needed to learn enough about crystallography to follow her work. He also needed to know what to look for in her X-ray photographs. Watson learned he needed to know if her pictures were consistent with a helical structure for DNA. Watson also hoped to collect ideas from Franklin's lecture that would help him and Crick develop a molecular model of DNA. In her lecture, Franklin said she believed the proper way to understand the structure of DNA was through careful work on X-ray diffraction and that building a model of DNA wouldn't work. She believed that using Tinkertoy models to understand the structure of DNA was a waste of time because only serious study of X-ray diffraction photographs would lead to an understanding of DNA's structure. Franklin said her work was preliminary but believed she would eventually understand the structure of DNA when she had collected sufficient X-ray diffraction photographs. After the seminar, Watson and Wilkins had dinner and discussed her lecture. Wilkins said he believed Franklin's recent work didn't advance their understanding of the structure of DNA, and he didn't believe she was photographing the proper parts of a DNA molecule to understand its structure. Wilkins also mentioned that his colleagues in biochemistry had given him samples of purified DNA, and he was able to produce X-ray diffraction photographs himself.

A few days after Franklin's lecture, Watson and Crick took the train to Oxford to meet Dorothy Hodgins and discuss her work on crystallography. On their way to Oxford, Crick asked Watson about Franklin's seminar. He specifically wanted to know the water content of the DNA samples she was using. Crick thought the water content of the DNA was important and began thinking about the problem theoretically. In a few minutes, he told Watson that only a few models were consistent with the results of Franklin's photographs and his own mathematical description of the alpha-helix. Crick began to draw a few simple models to show Watson how easy the problem of modeling DNA might be and how elegant the double helix structure was. Crick also said the X-ray diffraction data were consistent with two, three, or four strands of DNA, and they should study all three models. He also suggested that the angle and radii of the DNA strands twisted about its central axis would be critical to testing the model. Crick said that X-ray diffraction photographs would allow them to verify that their model was correct by comparing the angles and radii within the model with measurements from the X-ray diffraction photographs.

Crick said he believed they could develop their models fairly quickly and that comparing the models to the X-ray diffraction photographs would confirm whether they were correct. They continued to discuss possible options for the structure of DNA and decided that once the internal structure of the DNA helix was understood, the structure of the irregular base sequences might be obvious. They also agreed that the world's authority on structural chemistry was Linus Pauling, and they were at a serious disadvantage because he possessed a far deeper knowledge of biochemistry compared to them.[284] Moreover, Pauling had the training and intellect to solve the problem quickly if he applied himself and gained access to Franklin's X-ray diffraction photographs. Watson and Crick decided they needed to study biochemistry before they proceeded and set about looking for a copy of Pauling's book on the subject.

Biochemistry Text

They found a copy of Pauling's book *The Nature of the Chemical Bond* in Blackwell's bookstore in Cambridge and learned the proper sizes of the inorganic ions they believed were involved by studying his book, but still didn't know exactly how to construct their DNA model. When Watson and Crick went to work at Cavendish Laboratory the next day, their first task was to develop physical models of the atoms involved in a DNA molecule. They needed purine and pyrimidine bases (carbon and nitrogen compounds consisting of two rings fused together), but neither was available in the Cavendish Laboratory so they ordered them from the machine shop. Meanwhile, Watson improvised a way to build models by connecting copper wires to carbon atoms. He had trouble producing accurate physical models of the inorganic ions because they don't follow simple rules concerning the angles formed when making chemical bonds. Watson decided to work on other issues while he waited for the machine shop to finish making the purine and pyrimidine bases he needed to build his DNA models.

Model Building

Watson and Crick decided it might be more efficient if they worked on the general structure of DNA first and then tried to fit the inorganic ions into the general model later, so they began making a model in the form of a helix. Crick suggested they construct the simplest, most elegant model they could imagine because the best way to find DNA's structure was to follow Occam's razor (which says make no more assumptions than are necessary).[285] While Crick was thinking about the problem theoretically, Watson began constructing models, assuming the structure of DNA was a double helix. He believed that once he determined the positions of a few nucleotides, the resulting chemical structure would constrain the arrangement of other components, and he might be able to solve the puzzle with Crick's help. Over lunch, Watson and Crick discussed the most likely structure of the DNA chain and quickly discarded a "one-chain" hypothesis as inconsistent with the evidence. When they returned to the lab, however, they discovered that the model Watson had built didn't have the proper angles and distances required by the X-ray diffraction photographs, so he had to start over.

By the middle of the afternoon, Watson had constructed a model of the DNA molecule he thought looked promising because it seemed to fit the X-ray diffraction photographs. Watson and Crick contacted Wilkins and invited him to look at their model and tell them what he thought. Wilkins agreed and told them he would bring his colleague Rosalind Franklin with him for the meeting. Watson and Crick discussed how to share their work with Wilkins and Franklin and decided to proceed in two stages. First, Crick would discuss his helical theory, explain how their proposed model of DNA had evolved, and then adjourn for lunch. After lunch, they planned to discuss how they might proceed and propose a partnership with Wilkins and Franklin to study the structure of DNA through modeling.

Wilkins and Franklin Visit Cambridge

After Crick explained his helical theory to Wilkins and Franklin, Wilkins said he and Stokes had worked out the same basic idea weeks earlier. Rosalind Franklin disagreed with their idea of the double helix and became emotional, arguing that she didn't believe there was any evidence that the structure of DNA was helical. She said again that the solution to the structure of DNA would be found when she completed her work on X-ray diffraction rather than through modeling the DNA molecule with Tinkertoys. Franklin also told Watson he was incorrect in his recollection of the amount of water contained in DNA, so the model they had constructed was certainly wrong.

Watson and Crick were discouraged by her comments but felt they needed to reach an agreement with Wilkins and Franklin about how to proceed if possible. Franklin was not impressed with Crick's theory of the helix and said she intended to continue with her own work and was not interested in joining them. Wilkins appeared more reasonable, but they felt he was probably just trying to distance himself from Franklin rather than agreeing to work with them. Wilkins finally admitted he was not willing to work with Watson and Crick and left Cambridge. Watson and Crick decided to proceed on their own because that seemed to be their only option.

Sir Lawrence Bragg soon learned of the meeting among Wilkins, Franklin, Watson, and Crick and immediately let Crick know he must stop studying DNA, move on to something less controversial, finish his PhD thesis, and leave Cavendish Laboratory. Rather than follow Bragg's order, Watson and Crick simply kept a low profile and continued working on DNA without informing Bragg about what they were doing. They recognized that no more experimental data would be forthcoming from Franklin, and their model didn't fit the larger amount of water her work showed must be present in DNA. Watson had to start from scratch and develop a new molecular model. Both Watson and Crick were convinced that Wilkins and Franklin would not begin building models of a DNA molecule and they were at an impasse, so they worried that Linus Pauling might be the winner of the race to understand the structure of DNA if they didn't come up with a new model that fit the data fairly quickly.

Crick said he needed to begin working on his PhD thesis, and Watson agreed to look through biochemistry journals, trying to find a clue they had missed that would help them develop a model of DNA that fit the evidence. Crick gave Watson a copy of Pauling's *The Nature of the Chemical Bond* for Christmas, and he took that as a sign that Crick was still committed to building models of DNA with him. After Christmas, Watson and Crick learned that Pauling was coming to England and might visit Franklin to study her X-ray diffraction photographs.

Pauling's Work on DNA

When Watson learned that Pauling was planning to visit England, he was concerned the American would visit Rosalind Franklin, see her X-ray diffraction photographs of DNA, and be able to model the structure of DNA before he and Crick could build their own model.[286] However, the State Department saved them from that fate by withdrawing Pauling's passport because the US government believed he might say something controversial, such as criticizing a government policy, at a London news conference that would embarrass America.

Watson's friend and mentor Luria was also denied a passport to travel to England. Watson was asked to present the results of Luria's work on viral multiplication at a Society of General Microbiology meeting to be held at Oxford University. Luria told Watson he would send a letter explaining the work in detail, and Watson agreed to do the presentation. The letter noted that viruses infect other organisms by injecting their DNA into the host and that proteins didn't seem to be involved in the process. Watson believed this was good evidence that DNA was likely to be the primary genetic material rather than proteins, and he was delighted with this new fact because it reinforced his own belief that DNA was the key to understanding genetics.

Shortly after Watson returned from presenting Luria's research at Oxford, he was able to produce X-ray diffraction photographs that suggested the tobacco mosaic virus he was studying had a helical structure. The next day, Watson shared his X-ray diffraction photographs of the tobacco mosaic virus with Crick, who agreed that the structure appeared to be helical. Crick decided to concentrate on studying the molecular structure of DNA and neglect his thesis to help Watson. Watson continued reading the literature on genes and developed the idea that DNA was a template for making RNA chains, which then acted as templates for making complex proteins. Bad news arrived when they discovered Pauling had drafted a paper on the molecular structure of DNA and was ready to submit it for publication.

Pauling's DNA Paper

Watson learned from Linus Pauling's son, who was studying at Cambridge, that the American chemist believed he had discovered the structure of DNA. However, no further news of Pauling's discovery emerged, so Watson and Crick began to hope Pauling had concluded his theory was wrong or was waiting until he could obtain copies of the X-ray diffraction photographs Rosalind Franklin had produced before publishing. Watson discussed the fact that Pauling was working on the structure of DNA with Wilkins when he traveled through London later in the month, hoping Wilkins would ask Watson and Crick to join him in researching the structure of DNA before Pauling scooped them, but that didn't happen. When Watson returned to Cambridge, he learned from Pauling's son that his father had written a paper on DNA and would be submitting it for publication. Watson feared they had lost the race.

Pauling's son gave Watson and Crick a copy of his father's paper to study in detail. Pauling wrote that he believed DNA was a three-chain helix similar to the one Watson and Crick had proposed. However, after reviewing the paper, Watson realized that Pauling was wrong because the structure he was proposing was not an acid. All biochemists agreed that DNA was an acid, so Pauling's model could not possibly be correct. Crick also noted that the structure Pauling proposed didn't fit the X-ray diffraction photographs Franklin had produced. However, they both understood that once Pauling realized he was wrong, he would begin working to correct his error and probably discover the true structure of DNA fairly quickly. They had to begin working on their model immediately if they were going to claim the prize.

Wilkins and Franklin See Pauling's Paper

Watson traveled to London to discuss Pauling's paper with Wilkins and Franklin. Wilkins was busy when Watson arrived, so he went to Franklin's laboratory to see if she was available to discuss Pauling's paper. He gave her a copy of Pauling's paper and explained why he believed it was wrong. Franklin told Watson that DNA could not possibly be structured as a helix because her X-ray diffraction photographs offered no evidence to support that model. She then told Watson he would not make such silly mistakes if he took a serious look at her photographs and understood them. Watson replied that she was not competent to interpret her own photographs, and Franklin became angry at his remark. At that moment, Wilkins entered the laboratory looking for Watson, and Franklin calmed down. Watson and Wilkins left Franklin's laboratory to discuss Pauling's paper, and Watson told him he had been concerned that Franklin was going to strike him. Wilkins said that was possible because months earlier, Franklin had almost struck him when they had argued.

Wilkins Cooperates with Watson and Crick

The confrontation with Franklin and Pauling's paper changed Wilkins's attitude, and he began to share information about his work with Watson. Wilkins showed Watson new X-ray diffraction photographs he had taken that showed the molecule in a simpler way than the photographs Franklin had produced. Most important, Wilkins said the cross at the center of his photograph could only be the result of a helical structure for DNA. Watson recognized at once that with a copy of this photograph, he and Crick could measure the angles of molecules and calculate the number of chains in the DNA molecule. Wilkins said he believed Franklin's idea that the regular bases were located in the center of the helix was correct, but Watson and Crick thought the regular bases were more likely arranged on the outside of the helix. However, Watson and Crick still didn't have access to Franklin's X-ray diffraction photographs, and they needed them to complete their model.

Watson and Crick were at a standstill because they only had Watson's drawing of what he could remember of Wilkins's new X-ray diffraction photograph that he had prepared while returning to Cambridge by train. After studying the drawing of Wilkins's X-ray diffraction photograph, Watson began to wonder whether he should work on a two- or three-chain model of DNA. He decided to build a two-chain model of DNA because he believed all important biological things come in pairs. The next morning, Watson went to the laboratory to discuss what he had learned from Wilkins with Sir Lawrence Bragg. He made a sketch of Wilkins's X-ray diffraction photograph and explained the facts supporting their hypothesis that DNA was a helix. Bragg immediately understood Watson's argument and asked several relevant questions. Watson then told Bragg that Pauling was working on the structure of DNA and would likely solve the problem soon if he and Crick didn't begin working on the problem immediately. To his delight, Bragg told Watson to get on with the job of modeling DNA with Crick and beat Pauling to the prize.

When Crick came into the laboratory, Watson told him what Bragg had said and showed him the sketch of the X-ray diffraction photographs taken by Wilkins. Crick was excited about Bragg's statement, but skeptical of Watson's assertion that all things biological come in pairs. Crick believed the available evidence didn't allow them to differentiate between two and three-chain models and they should consider both. However, before they could begin building an accurate model of DNA, they needed the purine, pyrimidine, and phosphorus models from the machine shop and copies of the X-ray diffraction photographs produced by Franklin. While waiting for the machine shop to finish their order, Watson began putting together two-chain models of DNA, but none seemed right. Watson and Crick had a stroke of luck when they discovered that copies of Franklin's X-ray diffraction photographs were available in the files of a Cavendish

Laboratory committee established to supervise Wilkins and Franklin's work. With copies of Franklin's X-ray diffraction photographs in hand, they were able to solve the structure of DNA fairly quickly and build their molecular model.

Double Helix Confirmed

Once Watson and Crick were able to take accurate measurements from Franklin's X-ray diffraction photograph, they became convinced that the double helix model was correct. A few days later, Watson realized that hydrogen bonds could form between each of the four base pairs (adenine with adenine, cytosine with cytosine, quinine with quinine, and thymine with thymine). They hypothesized that DNA is written in the form of just four letters—A, T, G, and C (adenine, thymine, guanine, and cytosine)—which jointly control protein production. Their model of DNA suggested that gene replication begins when the two identical DNA chains separate and replicate, producing two new genes using half the original DNA pair as a template for each new gene.

Watson discussed his model with crystallographer Jerry Donohue at Cambridge, who told Watson he had used the wrong atoms in his analysis because the like-with-like structure would produce the wrong rotation of the helix and create too small an angle of rotation based on modeling Crick had done. Watson made cardboard models of the bases to work with until the machined purine and pyrimidine models arrived from the Cavendish shop. After trying various combinations of base pairs, Watson thought an adenine-thymine pair connected by two hydrogen bonds would be shaped the same as a guanine-cytosine pair held together by two hydrogen bonds. He then realized that hydrogen bonds would form easily and make the two shapes identical.

Watson believed the answer to DNA's structure was to assume that purine bonded to a pyrimidine. Pairing adenine with thymine and guanine with cytosine produced chains that were complementary and the pairs would be automatically determined. After playing with the cardboard models for a while, Crick and Watson decided the idea was plausible, but they needed to build a complete model using machined parts to verify that it satisfied the required three-dimensional chemical pairs and angles derived from the X-ray diffraction photographs of Wilkins and Franklin.

Watson went to the machine shop and persuaded them to finish the base pairs he needed. He returned to the lab, put the new machined base pairs into the model, and arranged them in what he believed were the correct positions. Watson began measuring the chemical angles to see if the model satisfied the X-ray diffraction data and the laws of chemistry.[287] After Watson finished checking the model, Crick examined it for about fifteen minutes and announced that he could find nothing wrong. They discussed how to make their discovery public and decided to check their model one more time before publishing to make certain they hadn't made an error. Watson and Crick used a plumb line and a measuring stick to determine the relative positions of atoms in their model. Once they were satisfied the model was correct, they invited Sir Lawrence Bragg to examine it. He understood the concept at once and saw how the pairing of adenine with thymine and guanine with cytosine produced the regular shape of a double helix. He advised them to have an organic chemist look at their work and verify that they had used the right formula and to discuss their model with Maurice Wilkins before they published.

Wilkins Verifies the Model

When Wilkins saw the model, he was impressed and offered to compare his X-ray diffraction data with the angles of their model. Wilkins said he would make the proper measurements on his photographs and let them know the results as quickly as possible. A few days later, Wilkins confirmed that his measurements were consistent with the DNA model that Watson and Crick had produced. They agreed that Watson and Crick, Wilkins, and Franklin should publish three papers simultaneously in *Nature*. When Pauling learned of Watson and Crick's breakthrough on the double helix model, the elegance of their DNA model convinced him that their idea was probably correct, and he graciously congratulated them. Watson and

Crick finished writing their paper and sent it to Wilkins and Franklin for comments. Sir Lawrence Bragg agreed to forward the three papers to *Nature* with a cover letter recommending the editors consider them for early publication.

Watson and Crick's article was published in 1953, and Francis Crick, James Watson, and Maurice Wilkins were awarded the Nobel Prize in Physiology or Medicine in 1962 "for their discoveries concerning the molecular structurer of nucleic acids and its significance for information transfer in living material."[288] Francis Crick died on July 28, 2004, in San Diego, California. James Watson served as a professor at Harvard before becoming director of the Cold Spring Harbor Laboratory from 1968 to 1994, when he retired. Later in his career, Watson was instrumental in managing and gathering funding for the Human Genome Project and received many honorary degrees from prominent universities.

Chapter 14

---- ✤ ----

THE HUMAN GENOME PROJECT: CHARLES DELISI

THE
HUMAN
GENOME
PROJECT

C ompleting the Human Genome Project involved collaboration among hundreds of scientists and funding from the National Institutes of Health (NIH) and the Department of Energy (DOE). Charles DeLisi first suggested mapping the entire human genome in the early 1980s, and James Watson (who jointly discovered the structure of DNA) helped convince Congress to fund the project. Senior leaders at NIH encouraged computer scientists to develop measuring instruments and computer programs to detect, sequence, store, retrieve, and analyze genomic data. The Cold Spring Harbor Conference organized by Watson generated scientific support for the project and helped persuade Congress to fund it. Having the entire human genome sequence available has produced significant medical benefits, including the identification of genetic mutations that cause cancer, the development of new medical treatments, the manufacture of genetically engineered biofuels, and the development of precise new tools for studying evolution.

Charles DeLisi was born December 9, 1941, in the Bronx, a borough of New York City. He attended DeWitt Clinton High School and graduated from the City College of New York in 1963. DeLisi worked as an engineer for the Sperry Gyroscope Company for two years before enrolling at New York University, where he earned a PhD in physics.[289] In 1972, DeLisi joined the Los Alamos National Laboratory to work on issues in theoretical biology.[290] After a few years in New Mexico, he became a senior scientist at the National Institutes of Health in Bethesda, Maryland, and joined the National Cancer Institute in 1975 to work on gene sequencing. Initial mapping of gene sequences was done by Walter Gilbert and Fred Sanger.[291] Their method allowed scientists to determine gene sequences but offered few insights into how genes actually worked, and the sequencing process was slow and tedious.

Constructing DNA Sequences

Another essential early step in sequencing the human genome was discovering a way to construct defined strands of DNA and combine them into longer sequences automatically. Kary Mullins discovered a way to manufacture short sequences of DNA automatically while he was searching for a way to copy DNA. After working on the problem for months, he tried using polymerase chain reactions (PCR) to perform the task.[292] Using PCR allowed Mullins to construct defined sequences of DNA and merge them into longer sequences automatically. Constructing genomic sequences was easier by using PCR to join smaller segments of genes into a longer sequence automatically. Using PCR simplified the process of replicating DNA, so gene sequencing progressed more quickly. However, the ability to organize and understand the information generated by these new ways of sequencing genes fell farther and farther behind because there were no automated databases or computer programs available to manage the data and allow scientists quick and easy access to the masses of genetic information being collected.

Before automated databases and computer programs were developed to store and analyze gene sequences, scientists estimated that sequencing the entire human genome would require a century using existing techniques because the process was so slow.[293] DeLisi was among the first to realize it would be possible to sequence the entire human genome more quickly and at lower cost if computer programs were available to identify genes, automatically recognize the sequence of amino acids involved, organize the sequences into databases, and analyze them to understand their biological properties.

Automated Gene Sequencing

Work on automating gene sequencing began in the late 1970s at the California Institute of Technology in Pasadena, California, one of the few institutions in America interested in structural molecular biology and the development of computer analytic techniques to automate biological processes. Henry Huang at Caltech was the first scientist to try automating DNA sequencing and developing a machine that could detect DNA segments. However, reliably detecting and differentiating DNA signals in a noisy background proved too difficult for him with the instruments and computers available at the time.

Lloyd Smith joined Huang at Caltech in 1982, and his knowledge of organic chemistry and measurement instrumentation helped them develop a way to detect DNA signals automatically. Hewlett-Packard and Applied Biosystems used Huang and Smith's results to link fluorescent dyes to DNA as marker signals and produce a reliable method of automating DNA sequencing. Applied Biosystems manufactured a prototype DNA sequencing apparatus and began selling it in 1987, but few genetic scientists were interested in using their apparatus. It was not until biologists became interested in sequencing the entire human genome that they realized how important automatically sequencing sections of DNA was and began using computers to organize and analyze genetic data. Biologists also had to discover how to construct known strands of DNA quickly.

DeLisi understood that genetic scientists needed a way to translate gene sequences into meaningful information quickly in order to understand the structure and function of the entire human genome. While at NIH, he supported applying machines to detect genomic sequences and computers to store and analyze the data to speed up the sequencing of genes. DeLisi helped develop the first automated gene-sequence databases, using computers and machines in learning to detect, analyze, organize, store, and retrieve genetic data. He believed that once automatic sequencing of genes was possible, scientists would become interested in sequencing the entire human genome.[294]

However, geneticists resisted applying computers to genetic sequencing because they didn't understand how machine learning and analysis worked or how they could be applied to answering basic genetic questions. DeLisi argued that developing machines and computer systems that could recognize basic DNA sequences and manipulate the four elements of DNA (the four chemicals adenine, thymine, guanine, and cytosine) the way computers recognize and handle 0s and 1s in computer code was an essential step in sequencing the human genome. He argued that automatic gene recognition and database management procedures had to be developed before the sequencing of the entire human genome would be feasible and cost-effective.[295]

Sequencing all forty-six chromosomes in a human cell was impossible using existing methods because each human chromosome contains millions of base pairs, and the total number of base pairs in the human genome is over three billion. When DeLisi first proposed using computers to analyze and sequence genes, only a few hundred thousand human genomic base pairs had been sequenced, and that had taken years. Sequencing three billion base pairs by hand would be impossible because the time and cost involved was prohibitive. It had taken years and the collaboration of many laboratories to map a simple yeast chromosome, and the human genome was thousands of times more complex. DeLisi argued that developing automatic genomic sequencing was essential to the Human Genome Project.

DeLisi asked Minoru Kanehisa, a computer scientist working at NIH, to begin developing a system to manage and analyze different databases, including DNA sequences, protein sequences, and the three-dimensional structure of proteins.

DeLisi and scientists at the Los Alamos National Laboratory also began working on a set of analytic tools that could automatically infer genetic functions and structural properties of DNA from their genomic sequences. Once these automated analytic techniques were developed, DeLisi believed the Human Genome Project could be successfully organized, funded, and completed. While work on these automatic analytic processes for sequencing genes was progressing within NIH, the Department of Energy asked DeLisi to join that agency as director of the Office of Health and Environmental Research (OHER). After careful consideration, he accepted the offer because it would allow him to manage larger and more complex projects involving computer scientists and geneticists. DeLisi believed that working at DOE would allow him to organize and fund more complex scientific projects and eventually interest genetic scientists in sequencing the entire human genome.[296]

Department of Energy

Once his security clearance was approved, DeLisi became director of OHER and assumed responsibility for managing programs in ecology, atmospheric science, epidemiology, and genetics. He soon realized he could not continue doing private research; his major focus had to be on administering the Department of Energy's budget, managing personnel, and lobbying Congress for funds. DeLisi committed to directing the organization because he believed that task would make a significant difference in the development of scientific policy. DOE was accustomed to funding large-scale projects other agencies were not equipped to handle. He set out to learn everything he could about the Health and Environmental Research Programs as it currently existed. Environmental research programs within the Department of Energy were conducted in laboratories at Argonne, Oak Ridge, Livermore, Berkeley, Brookhaven, and Los Alamos.

These laboratories were established to support the building of an atomic bomb during WWII.[297] DeLisi decided he needed to visit each laboratory personally, get to know the people, and discuss his plan for the Human Genome Project with them.

He was impressed by the quality and breadth of programs funded by the Department of Energy but felt almost overwhelmed by the amount of information he was collecting. DeLisi felt he needed to understand what was happening at each laboratory so he could fund them properly since he made the final decisions on who received grants. He was also concerned that Congress might not increase the budget for his agency over the next few years, so he set out to learn how Congress and the White House develop budgets so he could influence the process and receive money for the Department of Energy.

DeLisi was intrigued by a report from the Office of Technology Assessment about genetic mutations. In 1984, he received a report about the workshop held in Alta, Utah, that was drafted by the Congressional Office of Technology Assessment. The report contained ideas developed by leading molecular and human geneticists about how to detect heritable mutations. It concluded that detecting heritable human mutations would not be possible unless a large project was funded by the government for sequencing the entire genomes of parents and their offspring. DeLisi had been interested in developing just such a project to sequence the human genome before he read the article about the Alta, Utah, workshop authored by Renato Dulbecco and published in *Science*.[298]

The War on Cancer

Renato Dulbecco was president of the Salk Institute in San Diego and a Nobel laureate, so he was taken seriously by genetic scientists and members of Congress when he suggested that the War on Cancer would proceed more quickly if medical researchers could sequence the entire human genome. Dulbecco argued that if medical scientists wanted to understand cancer, they needed to study the entire human genome rather than just genes associated with viruses that caused cancers in animals. He wrote that when human cells change from their normal growth sequence to become cancer cells, there are detectible changes in the genetic structure of the cancer cells, and these changes might offer clues about how to cure cancer. He also argued that genetic changes in cancer cells could not be recognized or appreciated unless medical geneticists had access to a map of the normal human genome to use as a standard when searching for genetic changes in human cancer cells. Dulbecco's article outlining the relationship between human genome sequencing and the War on Cancer generated significant interest within the scientific community and government-funding agencies. It led to the convening of a conference at Santa Fe, New Mexico, to study the issue in detail.

The Santa Fe Conference

DeLisi wanted to know if it was economically and politically feasible to fund a program to sequence the entire human genome. His first step was to discuss the idea with several scientists to see if they were interested and would support the project. DeLisi wrote a letter to Mark Bitensky, a member of the Life Science Division at the Los Alamos Laboratory, asking if he would convene a workshop to discuss whether the Human Genome Project was a good idea and should be funded. Bitensky was excited about the idea and quickly organized a conference in Santa Fe, New Mexico, on March 3, 1986, which included many of the world's leading geneticists. Some were enthusiastic about the idea, but others believed individual scientists were already doing enough by sequencing sections of the human genome, and a large project would risk diverting funding from their important work. After extended debate, scientists at Santa Fe concluded that sequencing the entire human genome was technically feasible and would create significant progress in the War on Cancer.[299] They recommended that the Human Genome Project be national in scope, funded by several agencies, and managed by one.

Participants at the Santa Fe Conference suggested that the Department of Energy be given the lead role in organizing and managing the project because it had the experience and expertise needed to handle the job. It had developed and funded large projects such as NASA and knew how to organize a large bureaucracy. Finally, the participants at Santa Fe suggested that a scientific committee be established to advise the Department of Energy about strategies, administrative structures, budgets, and priorities for the project. DeLisi appointed Nacho Tinoco and Francis Collins cochairs of the committee responsible for guiding the project during its initial stages. Newspapers quickly broke the story of the Human Genome Project, suggesting that the Department of Energy was embarking on a project it was not qualified to manage and the research would cost several billion dollars, be impossibly complex, and would likely fail. DeLisi responded to this criticism by noting that the cost of sequencing the entire human genome would drop quickly as computational power and engineering expertise increased and the entire project would ultimately cost under a billion dollars.[300] James Watson took the next important step in bringing the Human Genome Project into existence by organizing a conference at Cold Spring Harbor to discuss its feasibility with genetic scientists.

Cold Spring Harbor Conference

In 1986, James Watson, codiscoverer of the DNA double helix, organized a meeting at the Cold Spring Harbor Laboratory on "The Molecular Biology of Homo Sapiens." The main topic at the conference was the possibility of sequencing the human genome. The Cold Spring Harbor meeting gave the project an intellectual and political boost because of Watson's reputation among scientists and members of Congress. The debate was heated because many young scientists were concerned that the Human Genome Project would siphon funding from their individual projects and stifle their careers. Others argued that science would become politicized, the project might not work, and NIH was already spending millions on gene sequencing, so why did they also need a giant bureaucratic project?

Scientists in favor of the project argued that genetic defects almost never involve just a few genes but are spread over several chromosomes and involve many genes, so having the entire human genome sequence available would advance our understanding of complex diseases such as cancer.

They also believed that the technology required to recognize and pinpoint defective genetic sequences could be developed from existing hardware, and the ability to rapidly sequence genes could be applied far beyond the War on Cancer or correcting genetic defects. At the end of the Cold Spring Harbor meeting, a majority of scientists was in favor of moving forward with the project proposed by DeLisi and the Department of Energy.[301]

The Cold Spring Harbor Conference stimulated a series of international discussions that attracted wide support within the scientific community. However, the project was seen as too ambitious by some younger scientists who argued that mapping the genetic sequences of simpler organisms should be completed before tackling the human genome. To deflect this criticism and attract additional support for the project, DeLisi proposed that physical mapping, linkage mapping, and sequencing of the chromosomes of simpler organisms be included in the Human Genome Project. He also proposed to support the development of analytic techniques to speed up the sequencing of genes and make the results cheaper to produce, more reliable, and more easily available before tackling the human genome.

DeLisi and Watson were instrumental in convincing scientists and the US government that mapping the human genome was desirable and feasible.[302] Once the project was authorized by Congress, genetic sequencing was performed at universities in the United States, the United Kingdom, Japan, France, Germany, and China. Charles DeLisi is usually given credit for originating the Human Genome Project, and James Watson was instrumental in convincing Congress to fund it. DeLisi and Watson agreed that the key to getting funding for the project was to convince Congress that the entire scientific community supported sequencing the human genome, so they approached the National Academy of Science directors to see if its members would publicly support the Human Genome Project before Congress if they were asked to testify. The National Academy of Science has a long history of advising the US government about science and was a key agency in convincing Congress to fund the project.

The National Academy of Science

President Abraham Lincoln signed a bill creating the National Academy of Science on March 8, 1863.[303] In 1916, George Hale, a prominent astronomer, wrote to Woodrow Wilson, suggesting that the president establish a National Research Council (NRC) to advise the government about scientific matters during wartime. The NRC eventually established standing committees to advise the government about funding for scientific research projects. In 1986, the question of whether the federal government should fund the Human Genome Project was submitted to the NRC for advice because its reports were respected by Congress. Bruce Alberts, a molecular biologist at the University of California San Francisco, chaired the NRC committee that discussed and made recommendations to Congress concerning the Human Genome Project.

Alberts focused the committee's early work on the scientific and technical aspects of the project and left the questions of funding for later. The committee members explored the science associated with the physical mapping of a genome, genetic linkage mapping, and somatic cell genetics before discussing the issues of computation, database management, and mathematical analysis of gene sequences. Another committee member, Maynard Olson at Washington University in St. Louis, had extensive experience in genetic sequencing from working on yeast chromosomes. He recommended the committee fund any project that was likely to increase the ability of scientists to sequence genes by a factor of three or more, and the committee members adopted his proposal. They eventually concluded that the Human Genome Project fit this criterion and decided to support it. They tasked a subcommittee with developing a proposed budget for the project and reporting back to the entire group with their recommendations.

The budget subcommittee presented three options: $50 million, $100 million, and $200 million annually for fifteen years. The National Research Council report supported the human genome sequencing program and recommended it be funded by the government with a budget of $200 million a year for fifteen years. The NRC report also established an agenda for the project and a proposal for use by Congress and the White House during their early budget discussions. The NRC report, published on February 11, 1988, recommended that a single governmental agency be appointed to lead the project, but didn't recommend whether that agency should be NIH or DOE.[304] Congress viewed the report as strong support for the Human Genome Project by the scientific community, and its members were generally favorable to funding the project. After the report by the NRC committee was issued, the new director of NIH became actively involved in managing the Human Genome Project and getting it funded by Congress.

NIH Director James Wyngaarden

The newly appointed director of NIH, James Wyngaarden, was instrumental in gaining congressional support for funding the Human Genome Project. He had been chairman of the department of medicine at Duke University Medical School and a well-respected clinician and geneticist before joining NIH as director. Wyngaarden, who represented NIH, and DeLisi, who represented DOE, met in 1986 to discuss the project and develop a joint plan for the two federal agencies to follow in dealing with Congress. Wyngaarden took the lead in managing and protecting the Human Genome Project budget from attacks by individual members of Congress who wanted to use research funds for their own pet projects, such as housing for the poor or expanding the Head Start program. However, the person who probably did more than anyone to convince Congress to fund the Human Genome Project was James Watson, codiscoverer of the structure of DNA, who was hired by NIH to lead the project in Washington, DC.[305]

James Watson

At a meeting in Boston in February 1988, NIH leaders asked James Watson, Nobel laureate and active genetic scientist, to lead the Human Genome Project, and he agreed. He recruited Elke Jordan and Mark Guyer to manage the project office in Washington, DC, and coordinate with other institutions around the country in managing the Human Genome Project.

As head of the Washington, DC, office, Watson helped NIH become the lead agency on the Human Genome Project because of his prestige in the scientific community and the respect he enjoyed among members of Congress. As codiscoverer of the molecular structure of DNA, Watson had a reputation for recognizing important research topics, and his support for the genome project helped assure its funding by Congress.

Watson guided the project during its formative years and made sure it had sufficient funding to sequence the entire three billion genes of the human genome over the next decade. His research ideas were considered "bold" and "intelligent" by geneticists and politicians, so they tended to follow his lead by supporting the project. After Watson's appointment to head the NIH genome project, staff from NIH and DOE met to discuss ways to cooperate and implement their memorandum of agreement. Committees were established by DOE and NIH to propose goals, ways to achieve them, and which agency would fund various parts of the project. Once they agreed on an agenda, both federal agencies began lobbying Congress for money.

Congressional Budgeting

DeLisi began developing the Department of Energy's budget for the fiscal year 1988 and planning how to gain support from the White House and Congress for the Human Genome Project. He decided to include a line item in the Department of Energy's budget for phase one of the project and rushed to meet deadlines because the DOE budget was due at the White House before January 1987, and it had to go through several review committees before that date. The White House Office of Management and Budget (OMB) elected to support the project and recommended that DeLisi include four million dollars in his first-year request for developing the engineering and computational infrastructure to support the sequencing of the human genome. Once he had agreement from OMB about the DOE's budget, DeLisi coordinated funding with NIH. However, DOE and NIH didn't always work well together because they had different cultures and expectations about how to manage a large scientific project.

The two federal agencies had different histories and reacted to the genome project in different ways. DOE was comfortable funding large technical projects that require a huge initial investment in instrumentation before the science begins because it had funded and managed NASA. In contrast, NIH was more familiar with funding smaller individual research projects directed by a single scientist or a small group of scientists that didn't require massive up-front expenditures for the development of technical hardware before the science began. The White House included funding for the Human Genome Project in the budget it submitted to Congress, but attitudes in the House and Senate were mixed about whether to fund it. DeLisi and Watson urged their colleagues at DOE and NIH to contact important scientists in the biomedical community and encourage them to support the project if they were called to testify before a congressional committee in hopes of getting adequate funding for their institutions.[306]

Getting support from President Reagan's administration for the Human Genome Project was only the first step. The next critical stage was to develop support within Congress, and that required cooperation from both agencies. However, many biologists had no idea the Department of Energy had been funding genetic research and paid little attention to it. However, Watson was well aware of the support the DOE had given to genetic research over the years, and when he called DeLisi to ask for a meeting, it was arranged quickly. When they met, it was clear to DeLisi that Watson was skeptical that DOE would be much help with Congress. NIH had requested funding for the Human Genome Project in its fiscal year 1988 budget, and Watson wanted DOE and DeLisi to lobby Congress to support funding for the project in testimony before the appropriation committee, and DeLisi agreed. After hearing Watson's arguments in favor of the project and DeLisi's support of it, Congress made funding available to both NIH and DOE to begin initial studies of computer programs to analyze genetic sequences and to develop an organizational structure for the project.

Congress appropriated almost $60 million to NIH and a little more than $25 million to DOE in 1990 for the Human Genome Project. The two agencies fought over funding for years before Congress eventually assigned NIH the role of lead agency on the project. During these years of conflict, David Kingsburg, head of the National Science Foundation, tried to mediate between the two agencies, which meant NSF could not compete directly for funding from Congress for the genome project. Once funding by Congress was assured and NIH was named the lead agency on the project, leadership at NIH and DOE shifted their focus from lobbying Congress to considering how to manage the Human Genome Project and organize the collection and analysis of data. They also needed to agree on a standard way to collect and organize the data.

Data Collection

To standardize data collected from the Human Genome Project, Maynard Olson, professor of genome sciences and medicine at the University of Washington and a specialist in the genetics of cystic fibrosis, suggested using sequence-tagged sites, which are short sequences of DNA that contain unique "tags" as reference sites on chromosomes.[307] Olson argued that using standard tags would allow different laboratories to communicate clearly and develop a standard language for discussing genetic sequencing. Using standard tags would also close the gap between physical and genetic linkage mapping and allow the mapping of individual genes.

Watson, as director, announced that the Human Genome Project would begin officially in October 1990, under the direction of NIH with funding from DOE and NIH. He suggested that the first few years should concentrate on planning, organizing, and developing computer programs and databases before the mapping of the genome began in earnest.[308] On July 11, 1990, the House Appropriations subcommittee held a hearing on the Human Genome Project to determine its current status and recommend future plans for NIH and DOE. The subcommittee meeting was the first public hearing attended by David Galas, successor to Charles DeLisi and newly appointed director of the DOE's Office of Health and Environmental Research. Watson and Galas both testified before the House Appropriations subcommittee, followed by the heads of several genome program research centers funded by DOE and NIH. Senator Domenici opposed the project because he wanted to cut the budget deficit and believed that taking money from basic research was popular with the public. However, his colleagues disagreed, and NIH and DOE secured increased funding for the genome project. The last undecided questions were how to apportion the money among various proposed projects, establish the organizational infrastructure needed to control the project, and begin building the engineering and computational infrastructure needed to manage the databases and analyze the sequences collected in later years. Getting genetic scientists interested in the automatic sequencing of genes using computers proved challenging.

Early Problems

Two problems surfaced during the development of computer infrastructure for genomic mapping: a lack of interest among biologists in computer and mathematical technologies to support genome mapping and too little money allocated for developing and managing databases using computer programs. However, when it was made clear to geneticists that the project would allocate funds to map the genomes of lower organisms as well as the human genome, these problems disappeared, and scientists began to realize that the focus of molecular biology was changing from small science programs to planned research projects. Scientists began to understand that automatic computer sequencing of the genome was essential before beginning to map the human genome because these automated computer techniques would make the mapping process faster and less expensive.

DeLisi and Watson

It's difficult to apportion credit for the Human Genome Project because DeLisi and Watson were both involved in developing the basic ideas underlying the project and garnering support from Congress to fund it.[309] DeLisi was more involved in convincing genetic scientists to support the application of computers to database management and analysis of genetic sequences. Watson had his biggest impact on the project during its early stages when he lobbied scientists for support, Congress for funds, and helped establish overall goals for research and development into the human genome. His research status attracted some of the brightest minds in biology to join the Human Genome Project and helped ensure its success. Watson resigned from the project in 1992 due to a long-standing disagreement with the new director of NIH, Bernadine Healy. He also opposed the patenting of DNA sequences and voiced his opposition before Congress, angering some scientists who wanted to profit from their work. Watson also raised serious ethical and moral issues concerning the Human Genome Project that angered some businesses but gathered strong support from scientists, government agencies, and Congress.

Ethical Issues

The primary ethical concern among scientists was how to keep insurance companies, employers, and other financially interested parties from discriminating against individuals who had genetic defects. Private citizens voiced serious concerns about patient privacy and the risk of discrimination against individuals based on genetic profiles and prenatal diagnoses that might uncover genetic defects and lead to abortions. They feared that being able to sequence individual human genomes would open a Pandora's box of ethical, legal, and religious issues involving genetic engineering and the risks of altering the human genome. To answer these concerns, Congress passed the Health Insurance Portability and Accountability Act (HIPAA) in 1996.[310] HIPAA was intended to keep individual health records from being released to unauthorized individuals or organizations, and the federal protection of medical records assured the public and most scientists that it was safe to proceed with mapping the entire human genetic sequence. The project proceeded.

A preliminary human genomic sequencing map was published on April 14, 2003, covering 99 percent of the human genome with an accuracy of 99.9 percent. By May 2020, the Genome Reference Consortium reported that many of the remaining gaps in the human genome had been filled, and a nearly complete sequence of the X chromosome was also available. Most scientists and politicians felt that the Human Genome Project had been a success and would bring many medical benefits in the future. By April 1, 2022, scientists reported they had filled all significant gaps in the human genome.[311] They identified many new genes that code for essential proteins and others whose function is unknown. They also corrected errors in an earlier reference DNA map and completed the $3 billion project. Finishing the entire map only cost a few million dollars because advances in computing technology had lowered the cost dramatically in the last decade. Scientists said that finishing the project felt similar to completing a gigantic jigsaw puzzle, and they predicted that the completed human genome would bring significant medical benefits to patients and physicians.

Medical Benefits

Having the entire human genome sequence available has already produced significant clinical benefits, including the identification of mutations that likely cause cancers, the development of new medicines, the manufacture of genetically engineered biofuels, and new tools for studying evolution. For example, the study of similarities among the DNA sequences of various organisms has allowed scientists to study human evolution in a new way. The human DNA sequence is available to any scientist with access to the internet and is located in a database labeled the GenBank. Computer programs are also available to analyze these data because it's almost impossible to understand the results of studies without significant analysis. The speed of these new automated gene-sequencing techniques is increasing at an exponential rate because of the development of more advanced computers.

Some interesting findings from the Human Genome Project include that the human genome contains approximately 22,300 genes, a number similar to other mammals, but the human genome has significantly more duplicated genetic segments than was expected before mapping was complete. Under 10 percent of human genes are specific to vertebrates, meaning that the vast majority of human genes are derived from other species, including lower organisms as far down the evolutionary tree as viruses. The entire human genome contains around three billion base pairs; but during the project, it was broken into approximately 150,000 smaller sequences, mapped separately, and then assembled into the entire human genome sequence.

To collect the initial genetic material needed to sequence the entire human genome, scientists working on the project took blood from several females and sperm from several males. Samples of this genetic material were selected for inclusion in the mosaic human genome that was eventually published. In this way, the identity of the original donors is protected so no one can learn their names.

Chapter 15

----- ✤ -----

GENE EDITING:
JENNIFER A. DOUDNA

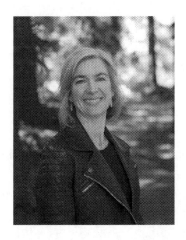

J ennifer Doudna was studying how CRISPR-associated enzymes borrow
bits of genetic material from attacking viruses and insert them into
the bacteria's own genes when Erik Sontheimer and Luciano Marraffini
reported that CRISPR-associated enzymes modify DNA rather than RNA.
They also suggested that CRISPR-associated enzymes might be used to
edit human genes and cure genetic diseases. Doudna immediately became
interested in developing a gene editing tool, decided she needed a colleague
to help her, and met with Emmanuelle Charpentier at a conference in Puerto
Rico. They agreed to collaborate and found that combining tracrRNA
and crRNA in a single sequence that contained a guide at one end and a

binding connector at the other allowed them to construct a gene editing tool. Doudna and Charpentier were awarded the Nobel Prize in Chemistry for their work in 2020. Gene editing has led to the successful treatment of inherited human diseases such as sickle cell anemia, Huntington's disease, and some forms of cancer. In the future, it may be possible to cure other genetic diseases using the tool.

Jennifer Doudna was born on February 19, 1964, in Washington, DC. Her family moved to Hawaii when she was seven. Doudna studied science and mathematics in high school and attended Pomona College in Claremont, California, where she earned a bachelor of arts degree in chemistry in 1985. She earned a PhD at Harvard University in biological chemistry and molecular pharmacology.[312] After finishing her doctoral degree, Doudna decided she needed to know how to produce X-ray diffraction photographs. She searched for a laboratory where she could learn the procedure and found one in Colorado.

University of Colorado

She contacted Thomas Cech at the University of Colorado because he had just won the Nobel Prize and could teach her X-ray diffraction. She asked Cech if she could do postdoctoral work in his laboratory, and he said "yes." Once Doudna learned how to crystallize RNA in Cech's laboratory, she tried using X-ray diffraction to study its structure but found that the solid RNA broke down. She discussed the problem with Tom Steitz, a young biochemist from Yale who was taking a sabbatical at Colorado, and he suggested she freeze the crystal RNA in liquid nitrogen to preserve its structure. The procedure worked, and Doudna published several articles on the structure of RNA. When she finished her postdoctoral fellowship, Doudna went to Yale University and continued working on RNA crystals.[313] She discovered that RNA has a defined three-dimensional shape before moving to the University of California in Berkeley.

University of California Berkeley

Doudna began working on how the RNA in viruses allows them to take over the protein-making machinery of host cells for their own use. She learned that CRISPR-associated enzymes in bacteria can borrow bits of DNA from attacking viruses and insert them into their own DNA so the bacterium can recognize the virus when it attacks again.[314] However, no one was certain how the process worked. While she was thinking about this problem, Jillian Banfield, a microbiologist at Berkeley said she wanted to meet with Doudna and discuss an idea she had developed. Banfield told Doudna she was trying to understand the purpose of CRISPR-associated sequences and wanted to work with someone who could analyze their molecular structure. Doudna thought understanding the structure of CRISPR sequences might be a fruitful approach to understanding how RNA interference worked and agreed to join Banfield.

They soon learned that RNA interference occurs when an enzyme called "Dicer" snips a long sequence of RNA into short fragments, and the short RNA fragments somehow locate messenger RNA that contains matching genetic letters and employs a process to chop up the matching messenger RNA. Doudna was intrigued by this finding and wanted to understand how it worked. She began exploring the molecular structure of Dicer by using X-ray diffraction crystallography and discovered it acts as a measuring tape after attaching itself to one end of an RNA strand. Next, she found that Dicer employs a scissor mechanism to slice the attached RNA segment to the correct length.[315] Doudna also discovered that she could replace an enzyme in the Dicer RNA sequence to generate a new Dicer that was able to slice and silence new genes.

At this point, Doudna decided she needed someone in her laboratory who had the skills and time to continue working on the project and began searching for a likely associate. Blake Wiedenheft contacted her, asking to work as a postdoctoral fellow in her laboratory; and when he discovered Doudna was interested in studying CRISPR sequences, he said that was a major interest of his as well. They began discussing possible research projects involving CRISPR sequences, and Doudna asked him to join her laboratory. She suggested Wiedenheft study the chemical components of CRISPR and concentrate on CRISPR-associated enzymes. Doudna recommended that Wiedenheft begin by studying Cas1, which appears in all CRISPR systems. Wiedenheft didn't know enough about X-ray crystallography to proceed, so Doudna suggested he work with Martin Jinek, an expert on X-ray crystallography, in her laboratory to learn the technique before studying CRISPR-Cas1.

Jinek decided that studying CRISPR-Cas1 with Wiedenheft was a good next step in his own research program, so they agreed to collaborate. Jinek and Wiedenheft constructed a three-dimensional molecular model of Cas1 fairly quickly. They found that Cas1 had a fold that could scissor genetic material from an invading virus and insert the material into the host cell's own genetic structure.[316] Then they learned that Erik Sontheimer and Luciano Marraffini had reported that Cas1 was modifying DNA rather than RNA, and that result opened a whole new area of study for Doudna and her research team.

CRISPR and Gene Editing

Sontheimer and Marraffini also suggested that it might be possible to develop a way to edit genes using the process.[317] They applied for a patent on the idea, but the application was rejected because they had presented no data showing how the process worked. There were several unknown factors that had to be defined before a functional gene editing system could be patented. Biochemists needed to study the basic components of CRISPR in the laboratory to understand the chemical process so they could control what was happening before it would be possible to edit genetic material. Sontheimer and Marraffini knew Doudna and her team had the biochemical skills and the experimental techniques necessary to understand the structure and chemistry of CRISPR sequences, and they called to see if she would be interested in working on the problem with them. Ordinarily, she would have been interested, but their timing was bad because Doudna was moving.

Genentech

In 2008, Doudna became interested in applied research that would help people immediately rather than do basic science that might have medical applications decades later. She was discussing her interest with representatives at Genentech, a genetic engineering company that had recently discovered how to produce synthetic insulin using genetic modification techniques. She was also discussing the company with former colleagues at Berkeley who worked at Genentech, and they told her it was a perfect place to do applied research. She accepted an offer from Genentech, but soon realized it was a mistake because she missed working on pure science.[318] Doudna returned to her former laboratory at the University of California Berkeley after two months' absence. She decided to spend more of her time mentoring young colleagues rather than only doing basic laboratory research.

Transitioning to being a manager happens in many fields: football players become coaches, writers turn into editors, and engineers move up to being team managers. A critical part of becoming a good manager is hiring the right people and then mentoring them, guiding their research projects, and helping them understand interesting experimental results. Doudna was good at finding bright young researchers who were self-directing; she liked mentoring younger colleagues and was able to help them understand the implications of their research findings. One of her first mentees was Rachel Haurwitz.

Studying CRISPR-Cas6

Rachel Haurwitz, a graduate student already working in her laboratory at Berkeley, fit perfectly with Doudna's mentoring plans. Doudna asked Haurwitz and Wiedenheft to work on a CRISPR-associated protein that was proving difficult to understand. They set to work and soon discovered that Cas6 had been entered into the scientific databases incorrectly, and that was why Doudna had been having so much trouble studying it. Once they found the correct sequence for Cas6, Haurwitz and Wiedenheft were able to produce the protein in their laboratory and learn how it worked. They found that Cas6 was attaching itself to RNA sequences generated by CRISPR and slicing them into short RNA segments that worked on an invading virus's DNA, confirming the work of Sontheimer and Marraffini.[319]

Their next step was to understand the structure of Cas6, but to do that, they needed help from Martin Jinek, the laboratory expert on X-ray diffraction crystallography. He agreed to join them on the project, and they found that Cas6 connects to DNA by finding the correct sequence and cutting it at a precise place without changing other parts of the DNA sequence. Moreover, only Cas6 of all the CRISPR-associated proteins seemed able to do that. Folds in the structure of DNA seemed to hold the key to understanding how Cas6 worked, but they didn't yet understand how the search-and-find mechanism functioned. The team appeared to be at a dead end and didn't know what they should do next when a new researcher joined Doudna's group at Berkeley.

In 2008, Sam Sternberg entered the PhD program at Berkeley to work with Doudna. When Sternberg first came to Berkeley, Haurwitz invited him to a party where they discussed CRISPR. Sternberg was intrigued by the conversation and told Doudna he wanted to work on CRISPR-Cas6 rather than RNA interference. She suggested he help Jinek understand how Cas6 worked. After attending a lecture by Eric Greene about single-molecule fluorescence microscopy, Haurwitz asked Doudna if he could go work with Greene to learn how to apply the technique to CRISPR-Cas6 protein. She agreed and he moved to Columbia to work with Greene. Sternberg published two papers with Greene, Jinek, Wiedenheft, and Doudna showing how CRISPR-associated RNA proteins find the correct sequence among the DNA of an invading virus so it can cut the critical sequence and insert it into the bacteria's DNA. They speculated that CRISPR-Cas6 was creating an immune system trigger in the bacterium in case the same virus attacked again.

A Gene Editing Tool

Doudna wondered if CRISPR-Cas6 could edit human genes and correct hereditary defects and decided to try developing and commercializing a simple tool that could be used in clinical laboratories to correct genetic defects in humans. She decided to create a start-up company to own the gene-editing tool, and Haurwitz agreed to form a private entity to commercialize basic research on CRISPR-Cas6 and apply it to medicine.[320] Haurwitz took courses at Berkeley's business school and became an expert on how to structure a start-up company, obtain and license patents, and commercialize basic research. She acted as president of the new company, and Doudna was the chief science adviser. While they were setting up their new entity, Doudna was contacted by a French scientist named Emmanuelle Charpentier, who had been studying CRISPR-Cas9 and wanted to collaborate on understanding how the CRISPR-Cas9 system worked.

Emmanuelle Charpentier

Doudna was interested in collaborating and agreed to meet Charpentier at a conference in Puerto Rico to discuss research on CRISPR-Cas9.[321] Charpentier had done graduate work at the Pasteur Institute in Paris on how bacteria become resistant to antibiotics and postdoctoral work at St. Jude Children's Hospital in Memphis on how antibiotics kill bacteria. After six years in America, she returned to Europe to head a genetics laboratory at the University of Vienna. By 2009, many researchers were interested in Cas9 after it was discovered that when Cas9 was deactivated in bacteria, the CRISPR system could no longer slice up an invading virus. This suggested to Charpentier that Cas9 was essential to the working of the CRISPR system and should be studied in detail. Scientists had also discovered that crRNA in bacteria contains genetic codes borrowed from viruses that had previously infected the organism, and crRNA seemed to activate Cas9 enzymes to attack a virus when it tried to invade the bacterium a second time. Charpentier was among several scientists interested in working on CRISPR-Cas9 as a possible gene editing tool.

CRISPR-Cas9

The CRISPR-Cas9 process Charpentier was studying involved a piece of RNA that acts as a template and an enzyme that can slice DNA. During her work with CRISPR-Cas9, Charpentier found that transactivating CRISPR RNA or tracrRNA was essential for CRISPR-Cas9 to work. She also learned that tracrRNA helped produce crRNA, the genetic sequence that remembers viruses, which had previously attacked a bacterium and acted as an entry point into the invading virus when the same virus tried to reinfect the bacterium. TracrRNA somehow allowed crRNA to find the correct spot on the invading virus for Cas9 to cut, which was essential for CRISPR-Cas9 to function properly.

Charpentier first began to suspect that tracrRNA was essential to the functioning of CRISPR-Cas9 when she found it was present in all CRISPR processes in bacteria. She was not certain what tracrRNA did but noticed it was always located close to CRISPR-Cas9, and she hypothesized it might be essential to how Cas9 worked.[322] To test her idea, Charpentier removed tracrRNA from a bacterium and found that the organism couldn't produce crRNA anymore. She speculated that tracrRNa controls the production of crRNA and put together a team to study exactly how tracrRNA actually works. Her team found that CRISPR-Cas9 accomplished virus recognition by employing tracrRNA, crRNA, and Cas9 enzyme. The process involved tracrRNA cutting long strands of RNA and transforming them into short crRNAs aimed at specific genetic sequences in the attacking virus.

In 2011, Charpentier and her team published their results in *Nature*. However, at that time, they didn't know exactly how tracrRNA functioned. To discover how tracrRNA worked and what it did, Charpentier needed to find a biochemist who could isolate the components of the tracrRNA process in a test tube and understand how each element worked chemically. That was her reason for meeting Doudna in Puerto Rico in 2011. As Doudna discussed collaboration on tracrRNA and gene editing with Charpentier, she thought of Martin Jinek, a biochemist and structural biologist in her laboratory who was looking for a new project and had the necessary X-ray crystallography skills to handle the challenge. Charpentier and Doudna agreed to work together and decided to add Krzysztof Chylinski, a Polish molecular biologist, to their team in addition to Doudna, Charpentier, and Jinek.

They were destined to make one of the most important discoveries in modern medical science: how CRISPR-Cas9 works and how it can be used to produce a gene editing tool for modifying human DNA. Charpentier and Chylinski met Doudna and Jinek in Berkeley to discuss ways to study how CRISPR-Cas9 works before returning to their respective laboratories in Sweden and Vienna to carry out the research project. The team arranged to hold regular remote conferences among Doudna, Jinek, Charpentier, and Chylinski to discuss problems, share ideas, and develop solutions to issues that arose. Their goal was to understand how CRISPR-Cas9 worked and create a simple and reliable gene editing tool using the process.[323]

Gene Editing

During their face-to-face meeting in Berkeley, Doudna and Jinek said they had been trying to make CRISPR-Cas9 work without success and were not certain why they were having trouble. After learning what they were doing, Charpentier suggested they include tracrRNA along with Cas9 and crRNA in their chemical mixture and see if that helped. When Doudna and Jinek followed Charpentier's suggestion, the three-element mix reliably sliced target DNA, and they immediately realized that tracrRNA was essential for crRNA to bind with Cas9. Next, they discovered that crRNA has a twenty-letter sequence that guides CRISPR-Cas9 to a DNA strand containing a gene sequence identical to the crRNA twenty-letter sequence. They also found that tracrRNA acted as a template holding the other elements in their proper positions while CRISPR-Cas9 attached itself to the target DNA. Once the connection between CRISPR-Cas9 and the target DNA (a defined genetic sequence within a genome) was accomplished, the Cas9 enzyme began cutting the target DNA at the proper site.

It was obvious to the team that a gene editing mechanism had important clinical applications in human medicine because different crRNA sequences could be created, used to find and edit any target DNA sequence, and the new crRNA would slice the target DNA at the proper place.[324] The gene editing mechanism they had discovered held the potential to change human evolution if applied early enough in an organism's development. They realized that by designing the correct crRNA, it would be possible to slice any DNA sequence and modify an organism's genetics. The team's next task was to find out if it was possible to make the CRISPR-Cas9 gene editing process simple and easy enough to employ in a clinical setting where it could be used to treat genetic diseases. They decided to see if they could connect tracrRNA and crRNA in a single sequence that would contain a guide sequence at one end and a binding connection at the other.[325]

Doudna, Charpentier, and their associates began by eliminating parts of the RNA sequences one at a time to see if CRISPR-Cas9 was still functional. Once they had reduced the RNA sequences to the minimum where it was still effective, they began searching for a way to connect the two sequences into a single RNA strand. While they were working on simplifying the gene-editing tool, Doudna's husband advised her to record what they were doing in a laboratory notebook, date the entry, and sign it before witnesses so she would prove patent priority at a later time if that became necessary. The team collaborated on drafting an article describing how CRISPR-Cas9 worked by sending copies to a Dropbox for editing by all four members. Doudna sent the finished paper to *Science* on June 8, 2012. The paper described in detail how crRNA and tracrRNA jointly connected the Cas9 enzyme to the target DNA and how the sequence contained in Cas9 determined where the slices would occur. The article also described how the team had fused crRNA and tracrRNA into a single strand RNA that could be used to edit genes.

The editors of *Science* realized they had an important paper on their hands, so they asked reviewers to return any comments on the article in two days to expedite publication. Doudna and Charpentier had discovered the critical elements of CRISPR-Cas9, showed how it worked, and developed a single-guide RNA—an important medical advance. *Science* accepted the article for publication on June 29, 2012, just three weeks after it was submitted and a few days before scientists were to gather for the annual CRISPR conference in Berkeley, California, to discuss the concept of gene editing.[326]

Competing Presentations

Doudna noticed that another paper was scheduled to be presented at the conference by Virginijus Siksnys of Vilnius University on how a Cas9 enzyme directed by crRNA was able to slice an invading virus. His paper had been rejected by several journals before Siksnys contacted Doudna, who was a member of the National Academy, and asked her to approve it for publication in the *Proceedings of the National Academy of Sciences*. She had just finished writing her own paper on the same topic, realized she had a conflict of interest, and recused herself from reviewing Siksnys's article. She did learn from the abstract of his article that Siksnys and colleagues had discovered several of the mechanisms underlying how DNA cutting is achieved by Cas9, and their paper suggested the results could be used to edit DNA. But there were gaps in their understanding of how the process actually worked, and Doudna believed her research was more complete.

Doudna's patent application and paper had been completed before she saw Siksnys's article. When he discovered what had happened, Siksnys acknowledged that Doudna had done nothing wrong by expediting the publication of her own paper and applying for a patent. That was how science worked—credit went to the scientist who published first. Siksnys and Doudna were both scheduled to present their papers at the CRISPR conference in Berkeley on June 21, 2012. However, priority for discovering the CRISPR-Cas9 gene editing process would ultimately go to Doudna's team because their paper had been accepted for publication on June 28, 2012, while Siksnys's paper would not be published until September 4, 2012, and Doudna's results were more complete.[327] Siksnys was asked to present his paper first at the Berkeley conference so he could receive some recognition for his independent work before Doudna's team presented their more complete explanation of how CRISPR-Cas9 works.

As Siksnys presented his findings, it became clear to Doudna that he didn't understand the essential role tracrRNA played in the CRISPR-Cas9 system, so it would be impossible for him to produce a functioning gene editing tool. After Siksnys finished his presentation, Doudna and Charpentier asked Jinek and Chylinski to present their findings because they had done the laboratory work and deserved the glory of disclosing their findings at the conference. Jinek and Chylinski were relaxed during their presentation because they were before a friendly audience, masters of the material, and had everyone's attention because their findings were considered important by everyone attending. Their presentation created a sensation. Everyone recognized that the work was original and fundamental to understanding how to edit genes.

Later that evening over dinner with Siksnys, Sontheimer, and Barrangou, Doudna discussed her plans concerning the CRISPR-Cas9 gene editing system. Siksnys asked Doudna if he should withdraw his paper, and she said "no." His team had made significant contributions to the field and should get credit for their independent work. Everyone understood they were in a race to apply the CRISPR-Cas9 technology to human genetic diseases and claim a patent on gene editing, which could be worth a fortune to the winner. The idea that genes could be edited was initially suggested by Paul Berg when he discovered what he called "recombinant DNA."

Gene Editing

The idea of editing a gene was first suggested in 1972 when Paul Berg at Stanford University discovered how to remove a small piece of DNA from one virus and splice it into the DNA of another virus.[328] Fifteen years later, researchers discovered how to transfer engineered DNA into mature human cells, but that type of DNA transfer was not able to modify human evolution because it didn't change a person's chromosomes. In 1990, physicians, using engineered DNA, inserted functioning copies of a missing gene into the T cells of a four-year-old girl who had a compromised immune system by removing T cells from her body, adding the missing gene, and then inserting the modified T cells back into her bloodstream. The functioning

T cells improved her immune system and allowed the child to live a normal life. However, she was not able to pass these modified T cells to her own offspring because the physicians had not altered her basic DNA.

Some physicians and researchers wondered if they could fix human genetic defects by editing defective DNA rather than simply adding a modified gene to mature human cells. However, this raised ethical questions about playing God and changing human evolution, and these first gene editing techniques, called TALENs, required a physician to create a new protein guide each time there was the need to slice a different DNA sequence. The procedure was difficult and costly. The advantage of the new CRISPR-Cas9 gene editing system proposed by Doudna was that medical scientists only had to construct the genetic sequence of the RNA guide, a simple task any competent medical clinician could do in an ordinary clinical laboratory. However, before CRISPR-Cas9 could be applied to human gene editing, it was essential to show that the system worked in a human cell that contained a nucleus rather than simply relying on chemical processes that worked in a test tube. Doudna entered the competition to patent the gene-editing tool with a handicap—no one in her laboratory knew how to work with human cells. Members of her team were experts in biochemistry, but the other teams in the race to patent the gene-editing tool contained experts who had experience working with human cells. Three major laboratories began working on the problem at the same time: Feng Zhang of the Broad Institute in Cambridge, Massachusetts; George Church at Harvard; and Doudna at Berkeley. The Church and Zhang teams had experience working with living human cells, which gave them an advantage in the race to develop a human gene editing tool.

Feng Zhang

Zhang became interested in genetic engineering in high school while participating in a gifted and talented program. He won third place in the Intel Science Search program and then enrolled at Harvard where he majored in chemistry and physics. Zhang went to Stanford for graduate study in Karl Deisseroth's laboratory, using light to stimulate neurons, map their brain circuits, and understand how the neurons worked. Zhang decided to follow up his interest in gene editing after he finished his PhD and applied for a postdoctoral fellowship to work with George Church at Harvard University to gain experience in gene editing.[329] Zhang joined the Broad Institute in Cambridge after publishing several gene editing studies with Church. He was already searching for a way to edit genes when he learned about CRISPR-Cas9. He was a late arrival in the field compared with Church and Doudna and didn't understand the essential elements of how CRISPR-Cas9 functions.

To remedy his lack of knowledge about how CRISPR-Cas9 works, Zhang contacted a graduate student in Church's laboratory who was working on CRISPR-Cas9 and suggested they collaborate. His friend from Harvard agreed to join the group. Next, Zhang contacted Luciano Marraffini, a postdoctoral fellow working in Sontheimer's laboratory at Northwestern University, who had experience working with human gene cells, about collaborating on CRISPR-Cas9 gene editing. Marraffini agreed to work with Zhang and suggested a way to make CRISPR-Cas9 work in human cells. Marraffini tested his idea on bacteria while Zhang tried the procedure on a human cell. Zhang was interested in developing a human gene editing tool when he read Doudna's paper and realized her team had solved the basic scientific problems of gene editing. All that remained was to show that her gene editing tool would work in a human cell, and Zhang and his team were already working on that process so they had a head start.[330]

In contrast, although Doudna wanted to apply her research findings on CRISPR-Cas9 to gene editing in humans, her team had no knowledge of how to culture human cells. Help came when Alexandra East joined her laboratory; she already knew how to grow human cells. By November 2012, Doudna's laboratory was finishing work on a human gene editing system using CRISPR-Cas9 when she received a call alerting her that George Church and Feng Zhang had each submitted papers to *Science* describing an RNA-guided gene editing technique for humans. Doudna gave Church a call, and he told her that *Science* had accepted both articles for publication. When Doudna asked Church if she should publish anyway, he said yes.

Race to Claim Priority

Doudna immediately called a colleague at Berkeley who ran an open-access electronic journal that accepted articles after a shorter review time than traditional journals. Jinek agreed to compile their experimental results and figures while Doudna wrote their article for the electronic journal. On January 3, 2013, *eLife*, the Berkeley electronic journal, accepted Doudna's paper for publication.[331] To add more drama, on January 29, 2013, another paper was published online showing that CRISPR-Cas9 worked in human cells. Four papers had been published on the topic in one month—Zhang, Church, Doudna, and a South Korean scientist named Jin-Soo Kim. In addition to competing for priority of publication, Zhang, Church, and Doudna were also racing to patent their findings.

To avoid a fight over who could claim priority for the patent, Doudna contacted Zhang at the Board Institute and Church at Harvard University and suggested they jointly form a company to license CRISPR-Cas9 gene editing. However, her proposal fell apart when she learned Zhang and the Board Institute had already been granted an expedited patent for using CRISPR-Cas9 as a human gene editing tool. Doudna and Charpentier had applied for their patent before Zhang but hadn't paid for fast-tracking, so Zhang was issued the first patent. Of course, this produced litigation.[332]

Patent Fight

The trial over who owned the original patent on human gene editing began in December 2016 before a three-judge panel of the Patent and Trademark Office in Alexandria, Virginia. The key issue was whether using CRISPR-Cas9 to edit genes in a human cell was obvious once Doudna and Charpentier had published their original paper in the *Proceedings of the National Academy of Science*. Zhang's attorney offered as evidence statements made by Doudna and Charpentier in their original article that it was uncertain whether their system would work in a human cell. Doudna's lawyer argued that these remarks were just signs of careful scientists, but his statement didn't impress the three judges, who decided Zhang's invention had not been obvious after Doudna and Charpentier published their paper. The patent judges decided Zhang owned the first patent. On appeal, the US Court of Appeals for the Federal Circuit held that Zhang was entitled to his patent, but that didn't preclude Doudna and Charpentier from receiving a second valid patent. The issue of who owned the patent on gene editing was unresolved although human gene editing seemed to have a bright future and lots of clinical benefits.

In early 2022, US patent authorities ruled that the Broad Institute deserved credit for inventing how to use CRISPR in plants and animals, effectively canceling the patent application made by Doudna and the University of California.[333] The 2022 ruling held that the University of California had failed to provide persuasive evidence they had produced a working gene editing technology for humans before the Broad Institute group received their patent. The patent officials reported that the University of California and its partners had the idea for a CRISPR-Cas9 gene editing system on March 1, 2012, but didn't show that their experiments were successful in plants and animals until after the Broad Institute team had been granted a valid patent.

Because more than one patent is involved and the legal issues still appear to be uncertain, legal authorities are recommending that if a company intends to become involved in gene editing, it should secure licenses from both the Broad Group and the University of California. Experts say the legal dispute makes no economic sense and the Broad Group and the University of California would be better off cooperating in developing the gene-editing tool, but neither side has been willing to compromise so far.[334] No matter who wins the patent fight, there are several promising areas where gene editing may improve human health.

Gene Therapies

Sickle cell anemia was an obvious candidate for gene editing because it is caused by a single-gene mutation. The CRISPR-Cas9 gene editing system is able to cure sickle cell anemia but is expensive (over $1 million per patient). Doudna and the Gates Foundation are searching for ways to lower the cost.

If they are successful, gene editing will offer real hope to over one hundred thousand Black children and adults who currently suffer from the disease in the United States.

Another promising application for gene editing is in the treatment of cancer. Chinese medical scientists have begun clinical trials of a few gene-edited cancer treatments, and US medical scientists are not far behind. The main way of attacking cancer through gene editing is to use CRISPR-Cas9 to disable a gene that produces PD-1, a protein that blocks the body's immune response to cancer cells. Preliminary reports from the University of Pennsylvania suggest the technique is safe but not very effective in treating cancer. There are also clinical trials in varying stages testing the efficacy of gene editing to treat leukemia, male pattern baldness, and elevated levels of cholesterol. Much of this work was put on hold in 2020 while scientists searched for ways to diagnose and treat COVID-19 before mRNA vaccines became available in 2021. Gene editing raises ethical, legal, and moral issues about human evolution.

Dangers of Gene Editing

Science fiction writers have warned for decades that modifying human genetics can have dangerous consequences.[335] Scientists and government leaders worry that creating superior genetically engineered human beings carries the danger of separating society into elite and ordinary human beings. Others argue that it is our duty to eradicate genetic diseases and improve the species and we shouldn't worry about changing human evolution for the better. A minority of scientists and government leaders believes gene editing should be banned before it creates a biological nightmare. Scientists are working on a set of ethical guidelines that will allow gene editing research to proceed under conditions that offer freedom to conduct research within certain limits so the procedure doesn't create bad unintended consequences.[336] These guidelines have provoked plenty of controversies and little agreement. When a Chinese scientist engineered a human baby, the world was outraged.

A Gene-Edited Baby

In 2017, He Jiankui submitted a medical ethics application to Shenzhen's Harmonicare Women and Children's Hospital to use CRISPR-Cas9 gene editing to modify embryos and allow couples suffering from AIDS to have babies who would be immune to the HIV virus. His procedure violated existing gene editing guidelines because it was not medically essential, but the hospital ethics committee gave him consent to proceed. Jiankui took sperm from the father, injected the sperm into the mother's egg, and implanted the fertilized egg in a surrogate mother. He injected CRISPR-CAS9 into the fertilized egg to delete the CCR5 gene from the fertilized embryo, allowed it to grow over two hundred cells, and then sequenced the embryo's DNA to verify that the gene edits had been successful. In November 2018, a surrogate mother gave birth by caesarian section to a pair of healthy females who possessed edited genes. The world's medical and scientific communities expressed serious concerns because Jiankui had not followed the ethical and legal guidelines established for editing the human germline. Jiankui was put on trial in China, found guilty, sentenced to three years in prison, and fined $430,000.[337] Doudna and Charpentier collected several prizes for discovering CRISPR-Cas9 gene editing.

Nobel Prize

The Breakthrough Prize in Life Sciences was awarded to Doudna and Charpentier in November 2014. On October 9, 2020, Doudna was awakened by a phone call from a reporter who told her that she and Charpentier had been awarded the Nobel Prize in Chemistry for their work on gene editing. The Nobel Committee stated that "this year's prize is about rewriting the code of life." The Nobel Committee excluded Feng Zhang and George Church from their award.[338] Before 2020, only five women had received the Nobel Prize in Chemistry among the 184 winners. Maria Curie, Irene Curie, Dorothy Hodgkin, Ada Yonath, and Frances Arnold had won the Nobel Prize in Chemistry before Doudna and Charpentier.

The main ethical concern with gene editing is the modified genes will change the course of human evolution. In the beginning, Doudna was against all editing of genes in embryos, but she has gradually changed her thinking. Today, she believes that decisions about gene editing should be left to individuals rather than dictated by scientists or governments. She also believes gene editing should only be used when it's medically essential and that engineering genetically enhanced children is morally wrong.

Conclusion

History of Medical Miracles explains the evolution of medicine through the biographies of physicians and scientists who made important discoveries. Medicine has moved beyond its primitive beginnings in magic and mysticism to a scientific understanding that diseases are caused by natural factors. The book examines early Greek and Roman medicine, human anatomy, blood circulation, germs, vaccines, antiseptics, X-rays, insulin, antibiotics, the structure of DNA, the human genome, and gene editing. Ancient Egyptian priest-physicians believed diseases were caused by angry gods or vengeful ancestors. In contrast, early Chinese physicians thought human health was regulated by the balance between yin and yang. Centuries passed before the Greek physicians Hippocrates and Galen concluded that human illnesses are caused by natural factors and began systematically studying the symptoms, courses, and cures for a few diseases.

Hippocrates

Hippocrates knew nothing of bacteria or viruses and could only speculate about the causes of disease, but he studied symptoms, treatments, and outcomes of illnesses and found effective cures for some diseases by trial and error. He believed human illnesses were caused by imbalances among yellow bile, black bile, blood, and phlegm and rejected mystical cures. Hippocrates is considered the father of modern medicine.

He rejected the idea that diseases are caused by gods or evil spirits, proposed that illnesses are caused by natural forces, recommended physicians carefully diagnose diseases, study their symptoms, record effective treatments, and apply that knowledge to help patients.[339] Six centuries later, the Greek physician Galen advanced the understanding of the disease by studying the anatomy of animals.

Galen

Galen believed that experience is the best source of knowledge, so he paid attention to treatments that worked. Galen also rejected the idea that illnesses are caused by angry gods and can be cured by prayer, arguing instead that diseases have natural causes and can be treated by observing which medicines, medical procedures, or surgeries work on illnesses. Galen studied anatomy by performing public dissections of living animals and demonstrated brain functions by pressing on different areas of an animal's cortex to show how pressure can cause temporary blindness or paralysis.

In AD 157, he was appointed physician to a school of gladiators and treated their wounds with oil, herbs, and wine to prevent infections. The alcohol and acidity in wine may have inhibited bacterial growth and promoted healing. He also believed the content of dreams could be used to diagnose illnesses.[340] Galen began his examination of a patient by collecting a physical and mental history, believing that past experiences and illnesses are essential to a proper diagnosis. He thought bleeding was not helpful if a patient was weak, young, old, pregnant, or when the weather was hot and dry. After his death, Galen became a medical legend because he championed the systematic study of disease. During the fifteenth century, his anatomical work was extended and corrected by Andreas Vesalius.

Andreas Vesalius

Attitudes toward science and medicine changed after the invention of printing in 1450, the discovery of America in 1492, the beginning of the Protestant Reformation in 1517, and Magellan's circumnavigation of the world in 1519. Natural philosophers began searching for knowledge by studying nature rather than relying on biblical authority. Vesalius was educated in this new attitude toward science and concluded that human dissection was the best way to study anatomy. He discovered that Galen, who was considered the world's authority on human anatomy, had made mistakes in his descriptions of the human body. Galen's anatomical work was based on animal dissections and contained serious errors. Vesalius taught anatomy at Padua Medical School and used illustrations, charts, human dissection, and an articulated human skeleton to demonstrate features of the human body during his lectures.

Around 1540, Vesalius began drafting an anatomy text based on his own dissections rather than the works of Galen.[341] His book contained seven hundred pages of text and two hundred illustrations of the human body. It was a publishing sensation due to the elegant illustrations, but its contents were not well received by the medical community because his findings contradicted Galen's teachings. Renaissance physicians believed the Greek physician was never wrong, and many rejected Vesalius's work. His academic career ended when Emperor Charles V appointed him as a household physician and ordered Vesalius to treat nobles and soldiers during his many wars. Approximately a century later, William Harvey discovered how blood circulates.

William Harvey

Galen believed veins originated in the liver, arteries originated in the heart, the liver produced blood that flowed back and forth in veins, and the heart worked like a bellows. Harvey showed that Galen's theory of blood circulation was wrong by dissecting human cadavers, performing elegant experiments on living animals, and observing how blood circulates in cold-blooded fish and shrimp. He built a private laboratory for studying and understanding human circulation. Harvey began his research by inserting a tube through the vena cava into the right ventricle of a human heart and injecting water, causing the right ventricle to swell. He noted that no water flowed from the right to the left ventricle of the heart, contrary to Galen's description of blood circulation. Through this one simple experiment, Harvey demonstrated that Galen's theory of blood circulation was wrong, but he still needed to understand the nature of circulation, so he devised several ingenious experiments to clarify how blood flows in the human body.[342]

He injected water into the vena cava and saw it flow through the pulmonary artery to the lungs. This suggested to Harvey that blood flows from the right ventricle of the heart through the pulmonary artery to the lungs and then back to the left ventricle of the human heart through veins for distribution to the body. He concluded that blood flows in one direction only and is moved by the beating of the human heart through arteries and veins. Harvey wanted to observe blood circulating in a living organism to verify his theory, but the hearts of warm-blooded animals beat too quickly for accurate observation. After an exhaustive search, he found a cold-blooded shrimp living in the Thames River that had a transparent body and a slow heartbeat. This animal enabled him to observe blood circulation through a magnifying glass. Harvey noted that blood flowed through the shrimp's arteries when the heart contracted, entered the right side of the heart via the vena cava, and when the heart contracted, blood was driven via the pulmonary artery into the brachia (the breathing organ of shrimp). At the same time, the contracting left ventricle of the heart pushed blood through the aorta to the rest of the body. Harvey believed he now understood human circulation but wanted to confirm his theory with further studies of mammals.

He observed that arteries dilated when the heart contracted, suggesting heartbeats cause the human pulse. He tested this idea by tying off an artery in a dog and verified that the pulse stopped in the artery beyond the ligation. In 1628, Harvey published his life work, *De motu cordis*, describing his experiments and theory of circulation. However, it took a generation before physicians accepted his findings about circulation because Harvey's work contradicted Galen's teachings, and the Greek physician was thought to be infallible. The next important advance in medical knowledge happened during the seventeenth century when a Dutch drapery dealer manufactured improved lenses and saw small organisms for the first time in water he collected from lakes and pools.

Antonie van Leeuwenhoek

Leeuwenhoek, an owner of a drapery shop, used magnifying lenses to judge the quality of cloth he purchased for his shop. He was dissatisfied with the lenses available and decided to manufacture his own. Leeuwenhoek created lenses that could magnify an object up to five hundred times but never revealed how he produced them. He was curious about everything and began collecting water from lakes and ponds to study under his microscope. He was surprised to see tiny creatures he called "animalcules" swimming in the water samples. Leeuwenhoek said the animals looked like tiny snakes, were smaller than a strand of hair, and came in various colors. He described his observations in a letter to the Royal Society that included detailed drawings of the small creatures he had seen.[343] The Royal Society asked their curator, Robert Hooke, to investigate Leeuwenhoek's claims because no one had ever seen such small creatures before. Using available magnifying lenses, Hooke was unable to see any small animals in the lake water. He had to manufacture a better lens to observe the small creatures Leeuwenhoek reported. Hooke showed his work to the fellows of the Royal Society, and they were impressed by Leeuwenhoek's discovery.

Leeuwenhoek saw other small organisms in a specimen he collected from a rotten human tooth but didn't connect the little creatures with tooth decay. He was even curious about how blood circulates. Although Leeuwenhoek knew nothing of William Harvey's work, he was able to verify Harvey's theory of circulation by observing blood flowing from arteries through tiny capillaries inside an organ and back through veins, confirming by microscopic observation the circuit that Harvey had speculated must exist. Leeuwenhoek also saw small animals produce more of themselves, disproving the theory that life develops spontaneously from filthy water. Up to that time, the theory of spontaneous generation was one theory explaining the origin of life. A century later, Edward Jenner discovered how to inoculate children against smallpox by exposing them to cowpox, saving millions of lives.

Edward Jenner

Around 1793, Jenner sent a letter to the Medico-Convivial Society reporting that children who became infected with swinepox seemed immune to smallpox. This is the first written suggestion that humans could develop immunity to smallpox by contracting a related milder disease. Jenner studied swinepox and cowpox for years, trying to understand how to transfer the mild disease from infected animals or children to healthy children to immunize them against smallpox. He collected and published fifteen cases of children who had contracted cowpox naturally and nine cases of children he intentionally infected with cowpox to prove that natural infection or intentional inoculation with cowpox protected children against smallpox. Jenner's early cowpox inoculations didn't always create immunity against smallpox, however, and he wondered why.

After experimenting with various methods of inoculating children, Jenner realized that the unreliable inoculations were caused by how he collected and stored cowpox serum. He discovered that only serum taken from a pustule between the fifth and eighth days after a child contracted cowpox effectively inoculated children against smallpox. Jenner believed that before the fifth day, the serum contained too little cowpox to produce good immunity, and after the eighth day, the cowpox had mostly disappeared. He also discovered that heating cowpox serum or storing the serum for several days caused it to be ineffective. Jenner was awarded a gold medal by the Royal Navy, voted ten thousand pounds by Parliament, and given an honorary degree of doctor of medicine by Oxford Medical School for his discovery of the cowpox vaccine.[344] His discovery led to the development of vaccines for many diseases including measles, mumps, polio, diphtheria, tetanus, pertussis, flu, and COVID-19. Also in the nineteenth century, William Morton discovered that ether had anesthetic properties that allowed physicians and dentists to perform painless operations.

William Morton

In 1844, while attending a chemistry class at Harvard College, Morton heard Professor Charles Jackson discuss the properties of ether and decided to see if the gas would act as an anesthetic and allow painless surgery. Morton began by administering ether to animals and then soaked a handkerchief in ether and inhaled the fumes himself. Morton felt lethargic, fell unconscious, and when woke, believed he could have extracted a tooth from a patient under the influence of ether without pain. He administered ether to patients to make certain it was safe and arranged a demonstration of the anesthetic to Boston surgeons. Dr. Henry Bigelow, a professor of surgery at Harvard Medical School, and Morton arranged a demonstration of ether as an anesthetic on October 16, 1846, in the operating theater at Massachusetts General Hospital.[345] After he recovered consciousness, the patient reported he had felt no pain during the surgery.

In 1846, Morton was granted a patent for his discovery of ether as an anesthetic. His former dental partner, Horace Wells, and Harvard professor Charles Jackson both claimed they had discovered the anesthetic effects of ether before Morton. However, Dr. Bigelow and other surgeons at Harvard Medical School disputed these assertions and supported Morton's claim of priority. Morton filed a request for compensation for his discovery with Congress but never received a dime even though a committee recommended he be paid. Morton served in the US Army as a surgeon during the American Civil War, using his anesthetic to operate painlessly on hundreds of wounded soldiers. During the middle of the nineteenth century, Joseph Lister began studying how to avoid surgical infections and saved countless lives with his discovery of antiseptics.

Joseph Lister

In the 1850s, some surgeons believed infections were caused by putting patients too close together in hospital wards. Other surgeons thought infections were caused by chemicals passing from one patient to another, and a few suggested that infections were caused by small organisms floating in the air. English surgeons knew infection rates were high in London hospitals, but no one was sure why. In 1852, Lister began studying what was causing hospital infections by collecting pus from infected wounds and looking at the samples under a microscope. He saw small creatures in his slides and wondered if they might be causing the infections. Lister learned about Pasteur's work on fermentation and spoilage of wine and speculated that hospital infections might be caused by small organisms in the air that were contaminating patients' wounds, causing infections and deaths. He decided to search for an antiseptic that would kill these germs before they killed his patients.

Lister began looking for a chemical that would kill the small creatures he saw in his microscope and found that dilute carbolic acid killed germs but didn't damage the surrounding tissue. He used carbolic acid on several patients with compound fractures and most recovered without developing infections.[346] Lister published his findings in *The Lancet*, reporting that he had developed a sterilization method based on Pasteur's theory of fermentation and germs. He recommended that surgeons bathe a surgical wound in carbolic acid to kill germs and avoid dangerous infections. Lister also calculated death rates at the Royal Infirmary before and after he introduced the use of carbolic acid during and after surgery. He found that the mortality rate dropped from 44 to 15 percent after he began using carbolic acid. Lister is best remembered as the surgeon who saved patients from hospital infections and pregnant women from infections following childbirth. Many surgeons continued to doubt that germs caused disease until Robert Koch found the specific bacteria that cause anthrax, tuberculosis, and cholera in the late nineteenth century.

Robert Koch

Koch began studying how germs cause illnesses after he read Pasteur's work on fermentation. Koch studied germs by collecting infected tissue from sick animals and humans for study under his microscope. In 1876, he first saw the germ that causes anthrax when a local farmer reported that his sheep were dying. Koch drew blood from a dead sheep, placed it on a slide to examine under his microscope, and found small rods and threads in the dead sheep's blood. He found that the rods and threads were always present in diseased or dead sheep, but never present in the blood of healthy animals.

Koch grew the small rods and threads in a test tube and found that they died when exposed to sunlight. He wondered how anthrax rods and threads were able to survive from one year to the next in a pasture but died when exposed to sunlight in his laboratory. Koch found the answer when he looked at a glass slide one day and saw that the rods and threads had turned into spores. He realized that anthrax survived in a pasture because it developed a protective coating when it turned into a spore. Koch recommended that farmers bury their dead sheep to prevent the spread of anthrax spores, and the procedure worked.

In 1881, he set out to find the microbe that causes tuberculosis. Koch collected tissue from a laborer who had died of tuberculosis and studied the infected tissue under his microscope. He saw nothing, so Koch decided to try using a stain to see if that would help him see the pathogen causing tuberculosis. He finally discovered that methylene blue dye allowed him to see tuberculosis bacilli.[347] They were much smaller than anthrax, but visible in his microscope when properly stained. On March 24, 1882, Koch presented his findings to the Berlin Physiological Society.

He proposed four rules to follow when trying to establish which germ is causing a particular disease: (1) to prove a microbe causes a disease, you must find it in every case of the disease but not in healthy cases; (2) the microbe must be separated from the diseased body and grown in a test tube as a pure culture; (3) the pure culture grown in a test tube must produce the disease when injected into a healthy animal; and (4) the same microbe should then be extracted from the new diseased animal and grown as a pure culture outside the body. Koch was awarded the Nobel Prize for Medicine in 1905 for proving human diseases were caused by germs. In the late nineteenth century, Wilhelm Roentgen discovered X-rays while experimenting with a cathode ray tube.

Wilhelm Roentgen

In 1855, Heinrich Geissler invented the cathode ray tube; and several years later, Roentgen decided to study Geissler's tube in his laboratory. He produced a stronger ray by increasing the electrical current passing through his tube. Roentgen discovered that the rays coming from his tube caused fluorescence more than a meter away while an ordinary cathode ray only traveled a few inches. Roentgen placed a piece of paper, a playing card, and a book in front of his vacuum tube and found that the fluorescence caused by the rays passing through a book was not so bright as the fluorescence caused by rays passing through paper or a playing card. He decided to test the ray with other materials and found that a thin sheet of aluminum diffused the rays about the same amount as a book, but a sheet of lead blocked the rays entirely.

Next, Roentgen decided to experiment with a small disk of lead by holding it between his thumb and finger to position it between the cathode tube and a screen. To his surprise, not only could he see the dark outline of the lead disk on his screen, but he could also see an image of the bones in his thumb and fingers! Roentgen had discovered a ray that produced an image of the human skeleton on a screen or photographic plate. During most of 1895, he worked on his new ray in secret to verify that it was repeatable and to determine if the new ray reliably produced an image of human bones on a photographic plate.

He submitted his results in a paper entitled "A New Kind of Ray" to the editor of the Physical-Medical Society and sent copies of the published paper to well-recognized physicists for comments.[348] Roentgen also enclosed X-ray photographs of his wife's hand and other objects to demonstrate the wide range of effects achieved with the "X-ray," as he called his discovery. Roentgen was awarded the Prussian Order of the Crown, Second Class, by the German kaiser, congratulated by eminent physicists, and given the Nobel Prize in Physics in 1901 for his discovery of X-rays. Roentgen's development of the X-ray ushered in a new era in medical diagnosis, allowing surgeons to see inside the human body to find where bullets were located, how bones had fractured, and to diagnose diseases of the gut and other internal organs. During the early twentieth century, Frederick Banting found a way to extract insulin from pancreatic tissue and use it to regulate the blood sugar levels of diabetic patients, saving many lives.

Frederick Banting

While preparing a lecture on carbohydrate metabolism, Banting decided to include a discussion about diabetes. During his preparation for the lecture, Banting began to wonder if secretions from the pancreas might be responsible for controlling blood sugar levels in animals and humans. He decided to isolate the secretion produced by the islets of Langerhans in dogs and see if the unknown enzyme could be used to manage diabetes. J. J. R. Macleod, an expert on diabetes, allowed Banting to work in his laboratory. In August 1921, Banting and his assistant, Charles Best, produced an extract from the islet of Langerhans that regulated blood sugar in a dog with no pancreas. However, making the extract was slow and expensive using their current methods, so they couldn't produce enough to treat the thousands of human patients suffering from diabetes. They needed a way to produce larger amounts of the extract efficiently.

Best and Banting tried producing the extract from fetal pancreatic tissue and found they could make more of the extract that controlled diabetes in dogs without a pancreas. To test whether it was safe to use in humans, Banting injected the liquid extract under his own skin and suffered no adverse reaction. Banting also found he could produce large quantities of the extract to manage diabetes from mature beef pancreas tissue. Macleod presented the team's results at a conference of the Association of American Physicians in Washington, DC, on May 3, 1922, summarizing their work and using the term "insulin" for the first time. He said insulin will treat human diabetes but warned that producing insulin on a large scale was difficult, and they needed to find a more efficient manufacturing procedure.

Best and Banting developed a more efficient method of producing insulin, and they signed a contract with Eli Lilly, a respected US pharmaceutical company to manufacture the drug. They also helped Lilly develop a way to produce large amounts of insulin at the company's plant in Indianapolis, Indiana. Clinical trials of the insulin produced by Lilly were successful, and it was approved for the treatment of diabetes by the US Food and Drug Administration.[349] In 1923, Banting and Macleod were awarded the Nobel Prize for their discovery of insulin. In 1928, Alexander Fleming discovered the antibiotic property of penicillin when he saw that a mold inhibited the growth of bacteria in his laboratory.

Alexander Fleming

Fleming recognized penicillin's ability to destroy bacteria in September 1928, when he saw that one of his culture plates had become contaminated with an unknown mold that inhibited the growth of bacteria. He grew the mold in beef broth and found that liquid from the mold killed the germs that cause scarlet fever, pneumonia, gonorrhea, meningitis, diphtheria, and strep throat. Fleming published his findings in the *British Journal of Experimental Pathology* in 1929 and continued trying to purify and manufacture the antibiotic for over a decade, with limited success.[350] In 1940, he read an article in *The Lancet* entitled "Penicillin as a Chemotherapeutic Agent," authored by scientists working at the William Dunn School of Pathology at Oxford University. Fleming visited Oxford, was shown around the laboratory, and told what the team was doing.

The Oxford group had discovered how to produce pure penicillin in larger quantities and tested the antibiotic in animals. They infected eight mice with streptococcus bacteria, injected four of the mice with penicillin, and left four untreated. The four untreated mice died in a few days while the four mice treated with penicillin remained alive and healthy. The Oxford team also tested penicillin on a human patient and found that it halted the growth of his staphylococcal infection. However, they ran out of penicillin before the patient was free of the bacteria, and he eventually died. The Oxford team traveled to America after proving penicillin was an effective antibiotic, hoping to find a US pharmaceutical company willing to manufacture the antibiotic for wartime use.

Merck, Squibb, Pfizer, and Lederle all agreed to produce penicillin for the US government. Penicillin production rose dramatically in the US and was released for civilian use late in 1943. On October 25, 1945, Fleming was awarded one-half the Nobel Prize for his discovery of penicillin; Florey and Chain at Oxford University shared the Nobel Prize for their work on purifying penicillin and showing that it was clinically effective. Fleming's discovery of penicillin lead to the development of several antibiotics over the next decades and saved millions of lives. After World War II, James Watson began studying the structure of DNA with Francis Crick at Cambridge University.

James Watson

In 1951, Watson was working in the Cavendish Laboratory at Cambridge, England, when he met Francis Crick. They liked working together and decided to try modeling the structure of DNA. Watson and Crick were aided by X-ray diffraction photographs of DNA produced by Rosalind Franklin and Maurice Wilkins. Watson and Crick believed they could find the structure of DNA by experimenting with physical models of DNA and comparing their models with measurements taken from the X-ray diffraction photographs produced by Franklin and Wilkins. They asked the Cavendish machine shop to make the chemical components of DNA so they could construct various molecular models until they found the correct one.

Crick suggested they assume DNA is a simple helix because any other structure would be more difficult to understand; and he believed the X-ray diffraction photographs were consistent with two, three, or four strands of DNA. They decided to construct the simplest model they could imagine, following Occam's razor, which says to make the fewest assumptions possible. Their early models didn't produce the proper angles and distances required by the X-ray diffraction photographs, so Watson and Crick collected precise measurements from Franklin's X-ray diffraction photograph before proceeding with building additional models. Watson decided that a double helix model was the most likely structure for DNA. He finally built a double helix structure that appeared to match the three-dimensional chemical pairs and angles derived from Franklin's X-ray diffraction photographs.

Watson began measuring chemical angles to see if his double helix model satisfied the X-ray data and the laws of chemistry. Once he and Crick concluded the model was correct, they asked Sir Lawrence Bragg to examine it. Bragg was impressed and advised them to discuss their model with Maurice Wilkins. When Wilkins saw the model, he offered to compare his X-ray data with the diffraction patterns derived from their model and confirmed that his measurements were consistent with the DNA model Watson and Crick had constructed. Francis Crick, James Watson, and Maurice Wilkins were awarded the Nobel Prize in Physiology or Medicine in 1962 "for their discoveries concerning the molecular structure of nucleic acids and its significance for information transfer in living material."[351] The next medical miracle required hundreds of scientists, a multi-billion-dollar budget, and a decade to complete.

The Human Genome Project

Charles DeLisi first suggested mapping the human genome in the 1980s, and James Watson helped convince Congress to fund the project.[352] The Human Genome Project required collaboration between hundreds of scientists and funding from the Department of Energy (DOE) and the National Institutes of Health (NIH). DOE and NIH began funding the project in 1984, and most of the human genome was mapped by 2003. The research was performed in the United States, the United Kingdom, Japan, France, Germany, and China. Senior leaders at NIH and DOE believed computers would be needed to store, retrieve, and analyze the masses of information produced by the project.

Charles DeLisi encouraged the development of instruments and computer programs to detect, sequence, store, retrieve, and analyze genomic data. Henry Huang at Caltech was the first scientist to study automated DNA sequencing using a computer. Hewlett-Packard and Applied Biosystems discovered a way to link fluorescent dyes to DNA as marker signals and developed a reliable method of automating DNA sequencing.

The Cold Spring Harbor Conference organized by James Watson generated support within the scientific community for the project, and Watson supported the project in his testimony before Congress. Because he had a reputation for recognizing important research topics, Watson's support persuaded Congress to fund the project. Having the entire human genome sequence available has produced significant clinical benefits, including the identification of mutations that can cause cancer, the development of new medicines, the manufacture of genetically engineered biofuels, and more precise tools for studying evolution. The final medical miracle involved editing DNA and has the potential to change human evolution.

Jennifer Doudna

Doudna was working on viral RNA when she learned that CRISPR-associated enzymes are able to borrow bits of DNA from attacking viruses and insert them into the bacteria's own DNA so it can recognize the virus the next time it attacks. At around the same time, Jillian Banfield, a microbiologist at Berkeley, told Doudna she was looking for someone who could analyze the molecular structure of CRISPR sequences using X-ray crystallography to map their shapes and find out precisely how they worked. Doudna said she was interested, and they agreed to collaborate. Erik Sontheimer and Luciano Marraffini reported that CRISPR-associated enzymes modify DNA rather than RNA and suggested it might be possible to edit human genes using the process. Their suggestion opened a new line of research for Doudna, but she needed a colleague to help with her work on gene editing.

Doudna met Emmanuelle Charpentier at a conference in Puerto Rico in 2011, and they agreed to study gene editing together. The CRISPR-Cas9 process Charpentier was studying involved a piece of RNA that acted as a template and an enzyme that could slice DNA. She had learned that transactivating CRISPR RNA (tracrRNA) was necessary for CRISPR-Cas9 to work because it helped produce crRNA, the genetic sequence that remembers viruses that had previously attacked the organism and acted as an entry point into the invading virus when it tried to reinfect the bacterium. TracrRNA somehow allowed crRNA to find the right spot on the invading virus DNA where Cas9 should cut and was essential for CRISPR-Cas9 to function properly.

To make a simple gene editing tool that could work in a clinical laboratory, Doudna and Charpentier tried combining tracrRNA and crRNA in a single sequence that contained a guide sequence at one end and a binding connector at the other. Once they had a single sequence containing both tracrRNA and crRNA that worked as a gene editing tool, Doudna and Charpentier began eliminating parts of the RNA sequence until they had reduced it to an effective minimum. Next, they connected the two sequences into a single RNA strand that could edit human genes. Doudna and Charpentier received the Nobel Prize in Chemistry for their work on October 9, 2020.[353] The Nobel Committee stated that "this year's prize is about rewriting the code of life." Before 2020, only five women had won the Nobel Prize in Chemistry among 184 winners. Their work has made possible the genetic treatment of inherited human diseases such as sickle cell disease, Huntington's disease, and some forms of cancer.

The Future of Medicine

Assuming that the current pace of medical discovery continues, effective treatments for cancer, dementia, and many genetic disorders may be near. However, there is no guarantee that medical research will continue to produce advances in treating human diseases. Today, medical scientists and government leaders face financial and ethical issues concerning the availability and distribution of modern medical care that need to be resolved. A serious issue is the uneven availability of quality medical care for the poor in rich nations, and a lack of basic medical care in poor nations. A major ethical issue involves how to balance patients' quality of life with the side effects of aggressive treatments for diseases such as cancer. Society and physicians have not developed a health care model that can deliver quality treatment to all citizens within rich countries, and there are no clear ethical guidelines for balancing quality of life with the harmful effects of aggressive medical treatments.

Moreover, many scientists are concerned that parents may want to genetically engineer superior babies, which could eventually create a race of elite humans. These social and ethical issues arise independently of progress in scientific medicine. Medical progress requires continued financial support for scientific and mathematical education, research, and the open sharing of ideas. Medical progress happens in fits and starts, triggered by careful preparation, hard work, and brilliant insights. Moreover, past progress is no guarantee that scientific medicine will continue to conquer human diseases in the future. Nature is unpredictable and microbes continually evolve into dangerous variants, so scientists must struggle to cure new forms of old diseases. Finally, because of the overuse of antibiotics in animals and prescribing them to treat viral infections, several diseases are developing antibiotic-resistant strains that require medical science to constantly develop new and more powerful antibiotics to kill these dangerous drug-resistant bacteria. It's not clear how long this process can continue before the bacteria gain ground.

However, human beings are naturally curious, and bright individuals over the centuries have worked to understand the world of medicine. They pushed the boundaries of scientific knowledge and medical practices by not being satisfied with the status quo. The future of medicine may contain more of these medical miracles if modern scientists continue to be curious.

Endnotes

1   Ancient Egyptian Medicine: Influences, practice, and magic. https://www.medical newstoday.com

2   The Placebo Effect: What is it? https://www.webmd.com. Pain Management

3   Definition of Traditional Chinese Medicine-NCI. https://www.cancer.gov.

4   A Chinese ivory carving of a doctor's lady. https://www.christies.com

5   Who Was Hippocrates? https:/www.livescience.com

6   Galen, Biography. https:/www.britannica.com

7   Andreas Vesalius, Biography. https://www.britannica.com

8   William Harvey, Biography. https://www.britannica.com

9   Antonie van Leeuwenhoek, Biography. https://www.britannica.com

10   Edward Jenner, English Surgeon. https://www.britannica.com

11   William Morton and the Painless Ether Anesthesia. https://scihl.org

12   Joseph Lister's antisepsis system. https://www.sciencemuseum.org.uk

13   Robert Koch, German Bacteriologist. https://www.britannica.com

14   Wilhelm Conrad Roentgen, Biographical. https://www.nobelprize.org.

15   Frederick G. Banting, Facts. https://www.nobelprize.org

16   Alexander Fleming, Biography. https://www.britannica.com

17   James Watson, Biography. https://www.britannica.com

18   Charles DeLisi. https://www.bionity.com

19   Jennifer A. Doudna, Facts. https://www.nobelprize.org

20   Medicine in the pre-Hippocratic civilization of ancient Greece. https://pubmed. ncbl.nih.gov

21   Ancient Greek Medicine. https://www.worldhistory.org

22   Of Gods and Dreams: The Ancient Healing Sanctuary. https://www.greece-is.com.

23   Hippocrates: The "Greek Miracle" in Medicine. https://www.ucl.ac.uk

24   Ancient Greeks: Everyday Life, Beliefs, and Myths. https://www.mylearning.org

25   Ancient Greeks: Everyday Life, Beliefs, and Myths. https://www.mylearning.org

26   Evolution of medical education in ancient Greece. https://journals.lww.com

27   The History of Anatomy. https://bodyworks.com

28   Hippocrates, Biography. https://www.britannica.com

29   Hippocrates, Biography. https://www.britannica.com

30 Hippocratic Method and the Four Humors. https://www.thoughtco.com

31 Differentiation of Fever, Greek Medicine. https://www.greekmedicine.net

32 The Plague of Athens. https://pubmed.ncbl.nlm.nih.gov

33 Hippocrates: The father of spinal surgery. https://pubmed.ncbl.nlm.nih.gov

34 What role did Hippocrates have in the history of epilepsy? https://www.medscape.com

35 The History of Dentistry. https://mikehambydds.com

36 The History of Dentistry. https://mikehambydds.com

37 Hippocratic Oath, Definitions. https://www.britannica.com

38 Galen, Biography. https://www.britannica.com

39 A Brief Look at Medical Student Syndrome. https://www.psychologytoday.com

40 Galen, Biography. https://www.britannica.com

41 Need Healing? You Need Aesculapius, Roman God of Medicine. https://www.icysedgwick.com

42 Galen, Biography. https://www.britannica.com

43 Roman Gladiator. https://www.worldhistory.org

44 Roman Baths. https://www.worldhistory.org

45 Galen, Method of Medicine, Volume III. https://www.loebclassics.com

46 The population of ancient Rome. https://www.cambridge.org

47 Titus Flavius Boethus. https://peoplepill.com

48 Roman Law and the Banishment of Dissection.https://94460593.weebly.com

49 Titus Flavius Boethus. https://peoplepill.com

50 Titus Flavius Boethus. https://peoplepill.com

51 Galen, On Diagnosis from Dreams. https://pubmed.ncbl.nlm.nih.gov

52 The Prince of Medicine: Galen in the Roman Empire. https://books.google.com

53 Marcus Aurelius, Biography. https://www.britannica.com

54 Antonine Plague. https://www.worldhistory.com

55 The theriac in antiquity. https://www.thelancet.com

56 Galen on the pulses. https://www.degruyter.com

57 A Brief History of Bloodletting. https://www.history.com

58 The Mysterious Death of George Washington. https://constitutioncenter.org

59 Galen's storeroom, Rome's libraries, and the fire of AD 192. https://www.cambridge.org

60 Galen, Biography. https://www.britannica.com

61 Andreas Vesalius, Biography. https;//www.britannica.com

62 Andreas Vesalius, Biography. https;//www.britannica.com

63 Andreas Vesalius, Biography. https;//www.britannica.com

64 Human cadaveric dissection: a historical account. https://www.ncbl.nlm.nih.gov

65 Andreas Vesalius, Biography. https;//www.britannica.com

66 Vesalius's Anatomy. https://www.bl.uk

67   Vesalius's Anatomy. https://www.bl.uk
68   Andreas Vesalius: Celebrating 500 years of dissecting nature. https://www.ncbl. nlm.nih.gov
69   A Brief History of Bloodletting. https://www.history.com
70   Andreas Vesalius, Biography. https;//www.britannica.com
71   Vesalius's Anatomy. https://www.bl.uk
72   Vesalius's Anatomy. https://www.bl.uk
73   Andreas Vesalius, Biography. https;//www.britannica.com
74   Andreas Vesalius, Biography. https;//www.britannica.com
75   Andreas Vesalius, Biography. https;//www.britannica.com
76   Andreas Vesalius' fatal voyage to Jerusalem. https://www.linkedin.com
77   William Harvey, Biography. https://www.britannica.com
78   William Harvey, Biography. https://www.britannica.com
79   William Harvey, Biography. https://www.britannica.com
80   History of the University of Padua Medical School. https://www.3decho360.com
81   William Harvey, Biography. https://www.britannica.com
82   William Harvey, Biography. https://www.britannica.com
83   William Harvey, Biography. https://www.britannica.com
84   William Harvey and the Discovery of the Circulation of the Blood. https://www. ahajournals.org
85   William Harvey and the Discovery of the Circulation of the Blood. https://www. ahajournals.org
86   William Harvey and the Discovery of the Circulation of the Blood. https://www. ahajournals.org
87   William Harvey: A Life in Circulation. https://books.google.com
88   William Harvey: A Life in Circulation. https://books.google.com
89   William Harvey: A Life in Circulation. https://books.google.com
90   William Harvey and the Discovery of the Circulation of the Blood. https://www. ahajournals.org
91   William Harvey and the Discovery of the Circulation of the Blood. https://www. ahajournals.org
92   William Harvey and the Discovery of the Circulation of the Blood. https://www. ahajournals.org
93   William Harvey's Anatomy Book and Literary Culture. https://www.ncbl.nlm. nih.gov
94   English Civil Wars. https://www.britannica.com
95   William Harvey, Biography. https://www.britannica.com
96   Antonie van Leeuwenhoek, Biography. https://wwww.britannica.com
97   Antonie van Leeuwenhoek, Biography. https://wwww.britannica.com
98   Museum of Microscopy. https://micro.magnet.fsu.edu

99   Who Invented the Microscope? https://www.livescience.com

100 Museum of Microscopy. https://micro.magnet.fsu.edu

101 Antonie van Leeuwenhoek, Biography. https://wwww.britannica.com

102 Antonie van Leeuwenhoek, Biography. https://wwww.britannica.com

103 Antonie van Leeuwenhoek, Biography. https://wwww.britannica.com

104 The discovery of microorganisms by Robert Hooke and Antonie van Leeuwenhoek. https://royalsociety publishing.com

105 How to Culture Infusoria for Baby Fish. https://www.ratemyfishtank.com

106 Galileo, Bibliography. https://www.britannica.com

107 Galileo, Bibliography. https://www.britannica.com

108 Antonie van Leeuwenhoek, FRS, and the Origin of Histology. https://lessonleeuwenhoek.net

109 Antonie van Leeuwenhoek, FRS, and the Origin of Histology. https://lessonleeuwenhoek.net

110 Antonie van Leeuwenhoek, Biography. https://wwww.britannica.com

111 Antonie van Leeuwenhoek, Biography. https://wwww.britannica.com

112 Antonie van Leeuwenhoek, Biography. https://wwww.britannica.com

113 Antonie van Leeuwenhoek, Biography. https://wwww.britannica.com

114 Edward Jenner, English Surgeon. https://www.britannica.com

115 Edward Jenner, English Surgeon. https://www.britannica.com

116 Edward Jenner, English Surgeon. https://www.britannica.com

117 Edward Jenner, English Surgeon. https://www.britannica.com

118 Edward Jenner and the Small Pox Vaccine. https://www.nclb.nlm.nih.gov

119 Edward Jenner and the Small Pox Vaccine. https://www.nclb.nlm.nih.gov

120 Edward Jenner and the Small Pox Vaccine. https://www.nclb.nlm.nih.gov

121 Edward Jenner and the Small Pox Vaccine. https://www.nclb.nlm.nih.gov

122 Edward Jenner and the Small Pox Vaccine. https://www.nclb.nlm.nih.gov

123 Edward Jenner and the Small Pox Vaccine. https://www.nclb.nlm.nih.gov

124 Edward Jenner and the Small Pox Vaccine. https://www.nclb.nlm.nih.gov

125 Edward Jenner and the Small Pox Vaccine. https://www.nclb.nlm.nih.gov

126 Edward Jenner and the Small Pox Vaccine. https://www.nclb.nlm.nih.gov

127 Edward Jenner and the Small Pox Vaccine. https://www.nclb.nlm.nih.gov

128 Edward Jenner and the Small Pox Vaccine. https://www.nclb.nlm.nih.gov

129 Edward Jenner and the Small Pox Vaccine. https://www.nclb.nlm.nih.gov

130 Edward Jenner and the Small Pox Vaccine. https://www.nclb.nlm.nih.gov

131 Woodville, William (1752-1805). https://www.oxforddnb.com

132 Edward Jenner, English Surgeon. https://www.britannica.com

133 Edward Jenner and the Small Pox Vaccine. https://www.nclb.nlm.nih.gov

134 Edward Jenner and the Small Pox Vaccine. https://www.nclb.nlm.nih.gov

135 Edward Jenner and the Small Pox Vaccine. https://www.nclb.nlm.nih.gov

136 Royal Jennerian Society for the Extermination of the Smallpox. https://collections.countway.harvard.edu

137 Edward Jenner and the Small Pox Vaccine. https://www.nclb.nlm.nih.gov

138 Royal Jennerian Society for the Extermination of the Smallpox. https://collections.countway.harvard.edu

139 Edward Jenner and the Small Pox Vaccine. https://www.nclb.nlm.nih.gov

140 Edward Jenner and the Small Pox Vaccine. https://www.nclb.nlm.nih.gov

141 Edward Jenner and the Small Pox Vaccine. https://www.nclb.nlm.nih.gov

142 Edward Jenner and the Small Pox Vaccine. https://www.nclb.nlm.nih.gov

143 William Thomas Green Morton, American Surgeon. https://www.britannica.com

144 History of Anesthesia. https://www.woodlibrarymuseum.org

145 History of Anesthesia. https://www.woodlibrarymuseum.org

146 History of Anesthesia. https://www.woodlibrarymuseum.org

147 Nitrous Oxide and the Inhalation Anesthetics. https://www.ncbl.nlm.nih.gov

148 William Thomas Green Morton, American Surgeon. https://www.britannica.com

149 William Thomas Green Morton, American Surgeon. https://www.britannica.com

150 Tarnisher Idol: William Thomas Green Morton. https://www.ncbl.nlm.nih.gov

151 William Thomas Green Morton. https://www.encyclopedia.com

152 History of Anesthesia. https://www.woodlibrarymuseum.org; William Thomas Green Morton, American Surgeon. https://www.britannica.com

153 William Thomas Green Morton, American Surgeon. https://www.britannica.com

154 William Thomas Green Morton, American Surgeon. https://www.britannica.com

155 William Thomas Green Morton, American Surgeon. https://www.britannica.com

156 William Thomas Green Morton, American Surgeon. https://www.britannica.com

157 William Thomas Green Morton, American Surgeon. https://www.britannica.com

158 William Thomas Green Morton, American Surgeon. https://www.britannica.com

159 William Thomas Green Morton, American Surgeon. https://www.britannica.com

160 William Thomas Green Morton, American Surgeon. https://www.britannica.com

161 Statements Supported by Evidence. https://.baumanrarebooks.com

162 William Thomas Green Morton, American Surgeon. https://www.britannica.com

163 William Thomas Green Morton, American Surgeon. https://www.britannica.com

164 An Appraisal of William Thomas Green Morton's Life. https://pubs.asahq.org

165 William Thomas Green Morton, American Surgeon. https://www.britannica.com

166 Joseph Lister Biography. https://www.britannica.com

167 Joseph Lister Biography. https://www.britannica.com

168 Joseph Lister Biography. https://www.britannica.com

169 James Young Simpson. https://www.rcpe.ac.uk

170 Joseph Lister Biography. https://www.britannica.com

171 Joseph Lister Biography. https://www.britannica.com

172 Crimean War. https://www.britannica.com

173 Joseph Lister Biography. https://www.britannica.com

174 Joseph Lister Biography. https://www.britannica.com

175 Joseph Lister and the performance of antiseptic surgery. https://www.ncbl.nlm.nih.gov

176 Joseph Lister Biography. https://www.britannica.com

177 Joseph Lister and the performance of antiseptic surgery. https://www.ncbl.nlm.nih.gov

178 Joseph Lister and the performance of antiseptic surgery. https://www.ncbl.nlm.nih.gov

179 Joseph Lister Biography. https://www.britannica.com

180 Louis Pasteur Biography. https://www.britannica.com

181 Joseph Lister Biography. https://www.britannica.com

182 Joseph Lister and the performance of antiseptic surgery. https://www.ncbl.nlm.nih.gov

183 Joseph Lister and the performance of antiseptic surgery. https://www.ncbl.nlm.nih.gov

184 Joseph Lister and the performance of antiseptic surgery. https://www.ncbl.nlm.nih.gov

185 Joseph Lister and the performance of antiseptic surgery. https://www.ncbl.nlm.nih.gov

186 Joseph Lister and the performance of antiseptic surgery. https://www.ncbl.nlm.nih.gov

187 Joseph Lister and the performance of antiseptic surgery. https://www.ncbl.nlm.nih.gov

188 How Victorian Doctor Joseph Lister and Antiseptics. https://www.npr.org

189 Joseph Lister and the performance of antiseptic surgery. https://www.ncbl.nlm.nih.gov

190 Joseph Lister and the performance of antiseptic surgery. https://www.ncbl.nlm.nih.gov

191 Joseph Lister and the performance of antiseptic surgery. https://www.ncbl.nlm.nih.gov

192 Joseph Lister Biography. https://www.britannica.com

193 Robert Koch biography. https://www.britannica.com

194 Robert Koch biography. https://www.britannica.com

195 Robert Koch biography. https://www.britannica.com

196 Robert Koch biography. https://www.britannica.com

197 Robert Koch biography. https://www.britannica.com

198 Cholera-Symptoms and causes. https://www.mayoclinic.org

199 Robert Koch biography. https://www.britannica.com

200 Robert Koch biography. https://www.britannica.com

201 Robert Koch biography. https://www.britannica.com

202 Robert Koch and the "golden age" of bacteriology. https://www.sciencedirect.com

203 Robert Koch biography. https://www.britannica.com

204 Robert Koch and the "golden age" of bacteriology. https://www.sciencedirect.com

205 Robert Koch and the "golden age" of bacteriology. https://www.sciencedirect.com

206 Robert Koch and the "golden age" of bacteriology. https://www.sciencedirect.com

207 Robert Koch and the "golden age" of bacteriology. https://www.sciencedirect.com

208 Robert Koch and the "golden age" of bacteriology. https://www.sciencedirect.com

209 Robert Koch and the "golden age" of bacteriology. https://www.sciencedirect.com

210 Robert Koch and the "golden age" of bacteriology. https://www.sciencedirect.com

211 Robert Koch biography. https://www.britannica.com

212 A Theory of Germs-Science, Medicine, and Animals. https://www.ncbl.nlm.nih.gov

213 The day we discovered the cause of the "white death." https://www.pbs.org

214 The day we discovered the cause of the "white death." https://www.pbs.org

215 The day we discovered the cause of the "white death." https://www.pbs.org

216 The day we discovered the cause of the "white death." https://www.pbs.org

217 Studies of tuberculosis and cholera of Robert Koch. https://www.britannica.com

218 Studies of tuberculosis and cholera of Robert Koch. https://www.britannica.com

219 Robert Koch-Tuberculin. https://www.museumofhealthcare.ca

220 Robert Koch-Tuberculin. https://www.museumofhealthcare.ca

221 Robert Koch-Tuberculin. https://www.museumofhealthcare.ca

222 Robert Koch biography. https://www.britannica.com

223 Robert Koch announces the discovery of a rinderpest vaccine. https://www.sahistory.org.za

224 Robert Koch announces the discovery of a rinderpest vaccine. https://www.sahistory.org.za

225 Professor Koch's Investigation of Malaria. https://www.jstor.org

226 Robert Koch biography. https://www.britannica.com

227 Robert Koch biography. https://www.britannica.com

228 Wilhelm Conrad Roentgen. https://www.britannica.com

229 Wilhelm Conrad Roentgen. https://www.britannica.com

230 Wilhelm Conrad Roentgen. https://www.britannica.com

231 Wilhelm Conrad Roentgen. https://www.britannica.com

232 Wilhelm Conrad Roentgen. https://www.britannica.com

233 Wilhelm Conrad Roentgen. https://www.britannica.com

234 Wilhelm Conrad Roentgen. https://www.britannica.com

235 Wilhelm Conrad Roentgen. https://www.britannica.com

236 Wilhelm Conrad Roentgen. https://www.britannica.com

237 Discovery of electricity. https://www.britannica.com

238 November 8, 1895; Roentgen's Discovery of X-rays. https://www.aps.org

239 November 8, 1895; Roentgen's Discovery of X-rays. https://www.aps.org

240 November 8, 1895; Roentgen's Discovery of X-rays. https://www.aps.org

241 November 8, 1895; Roentgen's Discovery of X-rays. https://www.aps.org

242 November 8, 1895; Roentgen's Discovery of X-rays. https://www.aps.org

243 November 8, 1895; Roentgen's Discovery of X-rays. https://www.aps.org

244 Max von Laue. German physicist. https://www.britannica.com

245 DETECTION OF SUBSURFACE DEFECTS USING E-RAYS. https://www.osti.gov

246 The Dangers of X-rays-Stanford University. https://large.stanford.edu

247 he Dangers of X-rays-Stanford University. https://large.stanford.edu

248 Wilhelm Conrad Roentgen. https://www.britannica.com

249 Wilhelm Conrad Roentgen. https://www.britannica.com

250 Sir Frederick Grant Banting. Canadian physician. https://www.britannica.com

251 Sir Frederick Grant Banting. Canadian physician. https://www.britannica.com

252 Sir Frederick Grant Banting. Canadian physician. https://www.britannica.com

253 Sir Frederick Grant Banting. Canadian physician. https://www.britannica.com

254 Sir Frederick Grant Banting. Canadian physician. https://www.britannica.com

255 Sir Frederick Grant Banting. Canadian physician. https://www.britannica.com

256 Sir Frederick Grant Banting. Canadian physician. https://www.britannica.com

257 Sir Frederick Grant Banting. Canadian physician. https://www.britannica.com

258 Sir Frederick Grant Banting. Canadian physician. https://www.britannica.com

259 Sir Frederick Grant Banting. Canadian physician. https://www.britannica.com

260 Sir Frederick Grant Banting. Canadian physician. https://www.britannica.com

261 Sir Frederick Grant Banting. Canadian physician. https://www.britannica.com

262 Sir Frederick Grant Banting. Canadian physician. https://www.britannica.com

263 Sir Frederick Grant Banting. Canadian physician. https://www.britannica.com

264 Alexander Fleming, Biography. https://www.britannica.com

265 Alexander Fleming, Biography. https://www.britannica.com

266 Alexander Fleming, Biography. https://www.britannica.com

267 Alexander Fleming, Biography. https://www.britannica.com

268 Alexander Fleming, Biography. https://www.britannica.com

269 Alexander Fleming, Biography. https://www.britannica.com

270 Alexander Fleming Discovery and Development of Penicillin. https://www.acs.org

271 Alexander Fleming Discovery and Development of Penicillin. https://www.acs.org

272 Alexander Fleming Discovery and Development of Penicillin. https://www.acs.org

273 Alexander Fleming Discovery and Development of Penicillin. https://www.acs.org

274 Alexander Fleming Discovery and Development of Penicillin. https://www.acs.org

275 Guns; not roses-here's the true story of penicillin's first patient. https://theconversation.com

276 Alexander Fleming, Biography. https://www.britannica.com

277 Alexander Fleming, Biography. https://www.britannica.com

278 Alexander Fleming, Biography. https://www.britannica.com

279 James Watson, Biography. https://www.britannica.com

280 James Watson, Biography. https://www.britannica.com

281 Franklin's X-Ray Crystallography. https://www.mun.ca

282 Linus Pauling-Biographical. https://www.nobelprize.org

283 James Watson, Biography. https://www.britannica.com

284 Linus Pauling-Biographical. https://www.nobelprize.org

285 Occam's Razon. Origin, Examples, & Facts. https://www.britannica.com

286 Linus Pauling-Biographical. https://www.nobelprize.org

287 James Watson, Biography. https://www.britannica.com

288 James Watson, Biography. https://www.britannica.com

289 Charles DeLisi-Biography. https://counterbalance.org

290 Charles DeLisi-Biography. https://counterbalance.org

291 Walter Gilbert, American biologist. https://www.britannica.com

292 Kary Mullins, American chemist. https://www.britannica.com

293 Charles DeLisi-Biography. https://counterbalance.org

294 Charles DeLisi-Biography. https://counterbalance.org

295 Charles DeLisi-Biography. https://counterbalance.org

296 Charles DeLisi-Biography. https://counterbalance.org

297 Manhattan Project. https://www.britannica.com

298 Renato Dulbecco, Italian-American virologist. https://www.britannica.com

299 Charles DeLisi-Biography. https://counterbalance.org

300 Charles DeLisi-Biography. https://counterbalance.org

301 Charles DeLisi-Biography. https://counterbalance.org

302 Charles DeLisi-Biography. https://counterbalance.org

303 National Academy of Sciences. http://www.nasonline.org

304 National Academy of Sciences. http://www.nasonline.org

305 Giants in genomics: James Watson. https://www.yourgenome.org

306 National Academy of Sciences. http://www.nasonline.org

307 Maynard V. Olson-National Academy of Sciences. https://www.nasonline.org

308 Giants in genomics: James Watson. https://www.yourgenome.org

309 Giants in genomics: James Watson. https://www.yourgenome.org; Charles DeLisi-Biography. https://counterbalance.org

310 HIPAA Privacy Rule. https://www.hipaajournal.com

311 Human Genome Map is Completed. Wall Street Journal, Friday, April 1, 2022.

312 Jennifer Doudna, Biography. https://www.britannica.com

313 Jennifer Doudna, Biography. https://www.britannica.com

314 Jennifer Doudna, Biography. https://www.britannica.com

315 Jennifer Doudna, Biography. https://www.britannica.com

316 Jennifer Doudna, Biography. https://www.britannica.com

317 CRISPR/Cas9 Targeted Genome Editing. https://www.umassmed.edu

318 Jennifer Doudna, Biography. https://www.britannica.com

319 Jennifer Doudna, Biography. https://www.britannica.com

320 Jennifer Doudna, Biography. https://www.britannica.com

321 Jennifer Doudna, Biography. https://www.britannica.com

322 Prof. Emmanuelle Charpentier, Ph.D. https://www.mpg.de

323 Jennifer Doudna, Biography. https://www.britannica.com; Prof. Emmanuelle Charpentier, Ph.D. https://www.mpg.de

324 Jennifer Doudna, Biography. https://www.britannica.com

325 Jennifer Doudna, Biography. https://www.britannica.com; Prof. Emmanuelle Charpentier, Ph.D. https://www.mpg.de

326 Jennifer Doudna, Biography. https://www.britannica.com; Prof. Emmanuelle Charpentier, Ph.D. https://www.mpg.de

327 Jennifer Doudna, Biography. https://www.britannica.com; Prof. Emmanuelle Charpentier, Ph.D. https://www.mpg.de

328 Biographical Overview, Paul Berg-Profiles in Science. https://profiles.nlm.nih.gov

329 Feng Zhang, Broad Institute. https://www.broadinstitute.org

330 Feng Zhang, Broad Institute. https://www.broadinstitute.org

331 Jennifer Doudna, Biography. https://www.britannica.com; Prof. Emmanuelle Charpentier, Ph.D. https://www.mpg.de

332 Patent Ruling Picks Winners in Fight Over Gene-Editing Tool. Wall Street Journal, Thursday, March 3, 2022.

333 Patent Ruling Picks Winners in Fight Over Gene-Editing Tool. Wall Street Journal, Thursday, March 3, 2022.

334 Patent Ruling Picks Winners in Fight Over Gene-Editing Tool. Wall Street Journal, Thursday, March 3, 2022.

335 The Dark Side of CRISPR-Scientific American. https://www.scientificamerican.com

336 The Dark Side of CRISPR-Scientific American. https://www.scientificamerican.com

337 Genome-edited baby claim provokes international outcry. https://www.nature.com

338 Jennifer Doudna, Biography. https://www.britannica.com; Prof. Emmanuelle Charpentier, Ph.D. https://www.mpg.de

339 Hippocrates, Biography. https://www.britannica.com

340 Galen, On Diagnosis from Dreams. https://pubmed.ncbl.nlm.nih.gov; The Prince of Medicine: Galen in the Roman Empire. https://books.google.com

341 Andreas Vesalius, Biography. https;//www.britannica.com

342 William Harvey, Biography. https://www.britannica.com

343 Antonie van Leeuwenhoek, Biography. https://wwww.britannica.com

344 Edward Jenner and the Small Pox Vaccine. https://www.nclb.nlm.nih.gov

345 William Thomas Green Morton, American Surgeon. https://www.britannica.com

346 Joseph Lister Biography. https://www.britannica.com
347 Robert Koch biography. https://www.britannica.com
348 Wilhelm Conrad Roentgen. https://www.britannica.com
349 Sir Frederick Grant Banting. Canadian physician. https://www.britannica.com
350 Alexander Fleming, Biography. https://www.britannica.com
351 James Watson, Biography. https://www.britannica.com
352 Giants in genomics: James Watson. https://www.yourgenome.org; Charles DeLisi-Biography. https://counterbalance.org
353 Jennifer Doudna, Biography. https://www.britannica.com; Prof. Emmanuelle Charpentier, Ph.D. https://www.mpg.de